MRCP1
BEST OF FIVE
PRACTICE PAPERS

Khalid Binymin

MBChB MRCP MSc
Consultant Physician and Rheumatologist
Southport and Formby General Hospital
Southport

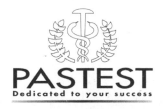

PASTEST
Dedicated to your success

© 2004 PASTEST LTD
Egerton Court
Parkgate Estate
Knutsford
Cheshire
WA16 8DX

Telephone: 01565 752000

First published 2004

Reprinted 2005

ISBN:1 901198 88X

A catalogue record for this book is available from the British Library.

The information contained within this book was obtained by the authors from reliable sources. However, while every effort has been made to ensure its accuracy, no responsibility for loss, damage or injury occasioned to any person acting or refraining from action as a result of information contained herein can be accepted by the publishers or authors.

PasTest Revision Books and Intensive Courses
PasTest has been established in the field of postgraduate medical education since 1972, providing revision books and intensive study courses for doctors preparing for their professional examinations. Books and courses are available for the following specialties:

MRCS, MRCP Part 1 and 2, MRCPCH Part 1 and 2, MRCPsych, MRCOG, DRCOG, MRCGP, DCH, FRCA, PLAB.

For further details contact:
**PasTest, Freepost, Knutsford, Cheshire WA16 7BR
Tel: 01565 752000   Fax: 01565 650264
Email: enquiries@pastest.co.uk   Website: www.pastest.co.uk**

Text prepared by Saxon Graphics Ltd, Derby
Printed and bound in Great Britain by MPG Books Ltd, Bodmin, Cornwall

CONTENTS

PREFACE

Most of the current medical examinations utilise the 'best of five' question format to assess doctors' knowledge and clinical experience. This book is comprised of four practice papers each with 100 questions. All questions are presented as real life clinical scenarios followed by five possible answers. The questions are new and cover all areas of medicine with special emphasis on topics that, from our experience, are more likely to appear in the MRCP examination. The questions have been designed to be brief and to the point. The answers are highly detailed, up-to-date and complete with authoritative medical explanations. The distribution of the topics in each practice paper is based on the MRCP part 1 syllabus outlined by the RCP guidelines.

This book should be regarded as a source of accurate and reliable information that will stimulate better understanding and fruitful interaction. It is very comprehensive and focuses on the very basics of medical principles and management. It will provide an excellent opportunity to test the reader's medical knowledge and help them gain a useful insight into the level of their preparations. The book is intended to satisfy the reader's needs and lift their standard and ability to answer the 'best of five' questions in a manner that will equip them to sail through future examinations with confidence.

I am greatly indebted to colleagues who reviewed this book for their generous help and criticism.

Good luck with your practice papers

Khalid Binymin

Acknowledgement

Julie Morris Msc., Head of Medical Statistics, Wythenshawe Hospital, Manchester

NORMAL VALUES

Blood, serum and plasma

Haematology

Haemoglobin	12.5–14.5 g/dl
Mean corpuscular volume (MCV)	80–96 fl
Mean corpuscular haemoglobin (MCH)	28–32 pg
Mean corpuscular haemoglobin concentration (MCHC)	32–35 g/dl
White blood cell count (WBC)	$4–11 \times 10^9/l$
Differential WBC: Neutrophils	$1.5–7 \times 10^9/l$
Lymphocytes	$1.5–4 \times 10^9/l$
Eosinophils	$0.04–0.4 \times 10^9/l$
Platelet count	$150–400 \times 10^9/l$
Reticulocyte count	$50–100 \times 10^9/l$
Prothrombin time (PT)	12–17 s
Activated partial thromboplastin time (APTT)	24–38 s
Thrombin time (TT)	14–22 s
Fibrinogen	2–5 g/l
Fibrinogen degradation products (FDP)	< 10 µg/ml
International normalised ratio (INR)	< 1.4
Iron (Fe^{2+})	14–29 µmol/l
Total iron-binding capacity (TIBC)	45–72 µmol/l
Ferritin	15–200 µg/l
Vitamin B_{12}	120–700 pmol/l
Folate (serum)	2.0–11.0 µg/l
Red cell folate	160–640 µg/l
Erythrocyte sedimentation rate (ESR)	< 12 mm/hour
Plasma viscosity	1.5–1.72 cP

Immunology/Rheumatology

C-reactive protein (CRP)	< 5 mg/l
IgG	6.0–13.0 g/l
IgM	0.4–2.5 g/l
IgA	0.8–3.0 g/l

Endocrinology

Fasting glucose	3.0–6.0 mmol/l
Hb A_{1c}	3.8–6.4%
Thyroid stimulating hormone (TSH)	0.3–4.0 mU/l
Thyroxine (T4)	58–174 nmol/l
Free T4 (FT4)	10–24 pmol/l
Parathyroid hormone (PTH)	0.8–8.0 pmol/l

Biochemistry

Sodium (Na$^+$)	137–144 mmol/l
Potassium (K$^+$)	3.5–4.9 mmol/l
Chloride	95–107 mmol/l
Urea	0–180 μmol/l
Creatinine	60–110 μmol/l
Calcium (Ca^{2+}), corrected	2.25–2.70 mmol/l
Phosphate	0.8–1.4 mmol/l
Creatine kinase (CK)	< 120 U/l
Uric acid	0–0.43 mmol/l
Copper	12–26 μmol/l
Caeruloplasmin	200–350 mg/l
Amylase	60–180 U/l
Alanine aminotransferase (ALT)	5–35 U/l
Aspartate aminotransferase (AST)	1–31 U/l
Alkaline phosphatase (ALP)	20–120 U/l
Lactate dehydrogenase (LDH)	10–250 U/l
Gamma-glutamyl transferase (GGT)	4–35 U/l (<50 U/l in men)
Bilirubin (total)	1–22 μmol/l
Total protein	61–76 g/l
Albumin	37–49 g/l
Cholesterol	< 5.2 mmol/l
Triglyceride (fasting)	0.45–1.69 mmol/l

Blood gases

pH	7.36–7.44
PaO$_2$	11.3–12.6 kPa
PaCO$_2$	4.7–6.0 kPa
Bicarbonate	20–28 mmol/l

Therapeutic drug levels

Digoxin ($\geq$6 h post-dose)	1–2 μg/l
Lithium	0.4–1.0 mmol/l

Urine

Albumin/creatinine ratio (random sample)	< 2.5 mg/mmol
Total protein	< 0.2 g/24 h
Glomerular filtration rate (GFR)	70–140 ml/min

Cerebrospinal fluid (CSF)

Opening pressure	5–18 cmH$_2$O
Total protein	0.15–0.45 g/l
Glucose	3.3–4.4 mmol/l
Cell count	< 5 cells/mm^3
Differential cell count: Lymphocytes	60–70%
Monocytes	30–50%
Neutrophils	None

Questions

PAPER ONE QUESTIONS

1 A confused 60-year-old man is brought by ambulance to the Emergency Department. His daughter tells you that he is a heavy smoker and that he has had repeated admissions with recurrent chest infections. She also says that her father has a chronic cough and can barely walk 100 yards before he has to stop because of shortness of breath. The chest X-ray shows hyperinflated lungs and right basal consolidation. Arterial blood gas analysis shows the following: Pao$_2$ 16 kPa, Paco$_2$ 9 kPa, pH 7.20. Which one of the following is indicated by the blood gas results?

☐ **A** Hyperventilation
☐ **B** The patient was given supplemental oxygen in the ambulance
☐ **C** Metabolic acidosis
☐ **D** That oxygen therapy at 60% and sedation should be instituted immediately
☐ **E** That the sample was venous and not arterial

2 A 60-year-old man was referred for further assessment of a cardiac murmur. On examination it was noted that he has a weak and slow-rising carotid pulse. The most likely underlying cardiac abnormality is

☐ **A** Aortic regurgitation
☐ **B** Alcoholic cardiomyopathy
☐ **C** Dissecting aneurysm
☐ **D** Hypertrophic obstructive cardiomyopathy (HOCM)
☐ **E** Aortic stenosis

3 A 60-year-old accountant complains of recurrent attacks of exquisite pain and swelling in the left big toe. Each of the following conditions is likely to be associated with this disorder, except

☐ **A** Chronic alcoholism
☐ **B** Obesity
☐ **C** Rheumatoid arthritis
☐ **D** Diabetes mellitus
☐ **E** Diuretic therapy

3

4 A 75-year-old woman is referred for assessment of her mental state. Her carer states that she noticed general decline in her physical and mental state. She is more forgetful and her concentration is poor. Sometimes her speech is incoherent. She trips frequently and had many falls. On rare occasions she has imagined seeing people sitting in her room. Each of the following features would help to distinguish between organic and functional disorders, except

- ☐ **A** Nystagmus
- ☐ **B** Visual hallucinations
- ☐ **C** Poor performance of the serial sevens test
- ☐ **D** Dysphasia
- ☐ **E** Hemianopia

5 You have been asked to see a 28-year-old librarian who is known to have schizophrenia which has been well controlled with anti-psychotic medications. She came with her friend and told you that she is feeling excessively tired and lethargic. Her friend added that she is avoiding going out and recently split from her boyfriend. She admits that she has lost pleasure in work, intimacy and even in sex. She has not had any auditory hallucinations or delusions recently. You referred her to see the psychiatrist. His report suggested that these symptoms are negative symptoms of schizophrenia and not depression as you had thought. Negative symptoms of schizophrenia include each of the following, except

- ☐ **A** Avolition
- ☐ **B** Affective flattening
- ☐ **C** Alogia
- ☐ **D** Anhedonia
- ☐ **E** Incoherence

6 A 30-year-old mechanic presented with central chest pain, worse on lying flat. He claims that he has had a flu-like illness for a week. Which one of the following ECG changes is most characteristic of this disorder?

☐ **A** PR prolongation
☐ **B** ST depression
☐ **C** Peaked, tall T wave
☐ **D** Prominent U wave
☐ **E** PR-segment depression

7 A 22-year-old woman has had four episodes of deep venous thrombosis. Laboratory studies should include each of the following except

☐ **A** α_2-Macroglobulin
☐ **B** Protein S
☐ **C** Protein C
☐ **D** Antithrombin III
☐ **E** Lupus anticoagulant

8 A 50-year-old woman has a history of gastrinoma and pituitary tumour. She reports increasing lethargy, drowsiness and constipation. The laboratory studies include raised calcium (2.9 mmol/l), low phosphate and raised PTH levels. The most likely diagnosis is?

☐ **A** Carcinoma of the bronchus
☐ **B** Pseudohypoparathyroidism
☐ **C** Acromegaly
☐ **D** Sarcoidosis
☐ **E** Multiple endocrine neoplasia syndrome (MEN I)

9   A 58-year-old man was admitted with a three-weeks history of
    shortness of breath. The chest X-ray demonstrates a right pleural
    effusion. Pleural fluid analysis shows 6600 mm³ WBC,
    40% eosinophils. The condition least likely to be responsible for
    this clinical presentation is

    ☐   A   Pneumothorax
    ☐   B   Haemothorax
    ☐   C   Pulmonary infarction
    ☐   D   Benign asbestos pleural effusion
    ☐   E   Tuberculous pleural effusion

10 A 60-year-old teacher is being investigated for increasing
    shortness of breath and diffuse fibrotic changes found on plain
    chest X-rays. He was taking diuretics and anti-arrhythmic
    treatment. The 12-lead ECG shows a prolonged QT interval. Each
    of the following clinical situations could be responsible for this
    ECG abnormality, except

    ☐   A   Heart failure
    ☐   B   Hypokalaemia
    ☐   C   Furosemide therapy
    ☐   D   Hypercalcaemia
    ☐   E   Amiodarone therapy

11 A 20-year-old woman is referred for further investigation. She
    gave a history of three episodes of meningitis proved to be due
    to recurrent meningococcal infections. Deficiency of which of
    the complement system factors is responsible for increased
    susceptibility to this infection?

    ☐   A   C3
    ☐   B   C1 esterase inhibitor
    ☐   C   C8
    ☐   D   C1q
    ☐   E   C2

12 A 56-year-old man has had sinusitis for a few months. Recently he complained of bloody nasal discharge, cough, and shortness of breath. The chest X-ray shows a diffuse area of consolidation and cavities in the right middle lobe and left upper lobe. Urinalysis shows red blood casts and protein ++++. The most likely diagnosis is

- [ ] **A** Aspiration pneumonia
- [ ] **B** Pulmonary tuberculosis
- [ ] **C** Carcinoma of the bronchus
- [x] **D** Wegener's granulomatosis
- [ ] **E** Sarcoidosis

13 A 37-year-old farmer with a one-year history of epilepsy is referred for further assessment. A CT scan of the brain shows several space-occupying cystic lesions throughout the brain. A serum specimen was positive for cysticercosis by immunoblot assay. The patient most likely acquired this disease by eating which one of the following types of poorly cooked food?

- [ ] **A** Chicken
- [ ] **B** Beef
- [ ] **C** Pork
- [ ] **D** Fish
- [ ] **E** Snails

14 A 25-year-old university lecturer with a history of asthma and nasal polyp has recurrent episodes of dyspnoea and cough whenever she takes aspirin. She should be advised to avoid taking which one of the following medications?

- [ ] **A** Paracetamol
- [ ] **B** Diclofenac sodium
- [ ] **C** Codeine
- [ ] **D** Ranitidine
- [ ] **E** Trimethoprim

15 A 40-year-old butcher complains of pain and paraesthesia in both hands. On examination he has wasting of the right thenar muscles, and tapping the volar aspect of the right wrist provoked a pins and needle sensation in the index and middle finger. Each of the following disorders could be responsible for the clinical features, except

☐ A Hypothyroidism
☐ B Acromegaly
☐ C Rheumatoid arthritis
☐ D Diabetes mellitus
☐ E Haemochromatosis

16 In a 22-year-old student with hypertrophic obstructive cardiomyopathy (HOCM) the most likely description of the carotid pulse is

☐ A Slow-rising carotid pulse
☐ B A bisferious carotid pulse
☐ C Pulsus paradoxus
☐ D A 'spike and dome' carotid pulse
☐ E A dicrotic carotid pulse

17 A 65-year-old accountant complains of exquisite pain in the left loin. Ultrasound of the kidneys confirms the presence of two renal calculi in the left kidney. In the last two years he has had three attacks of acute arthritis affecting the big toe, each lasting for a week or two before complete recovery. Which one of the following statements is not true about this disorder?

☐ A Pethidine is very useful in controlling severe renal colic
☐ B Urine acidity promotes nephrolithiasis
☐ C Allopurinol therapy should be initiated
☐ D Calcium oxalate stones are the most likely cause of the renal colic
☐ E Colchicine is of value in reducing the frequency of recurrent acute gouty arthritis

18 A 55-year-old man was referred because he has shortness of breath after minimal exertion, and non-productive cough. These symptoms started nine months earlier and were not preceded by any febrile illness. He smoked heavily during most of his adult life. Physical examination revealed fine crepitations in mid- and lower zones and clubbing of the fingers. The most likely diagnosis is

☐ A Pulmonary tuberculosis (TB)
☐ B Carcinoma of the bronchus
☐ C Bronchiectasis
☐ D Fibrosing alveolitis
☐ E Chronic obstructive pulmonary disease

19 A 45-year-old man was referred with impotence, hypogonadism, raised ALT, and arthritis affecting the second and third metatarsophalangeal joints. The most likely diagnosis is

☐ A Haemochromatosis
☐ B Diabetes mellitus
☐ C Brain tumour
☐ D Wilson's disease
☐ E Acromegaly

20 A 25-year-old man is referred for evaluation of infertility. Physical examination reveals a tall, obese man with bilateral gynaecomastia and small, firm testes. Which of the following is the most appropriate test to establish the cause of this man's infertility?

☐ A Semen analysis
☐ B Testicular biopsy
☐ C Serum testosterone
☐ D Magnetic resonance imaging (MRI) of the sella turcica
☐ E Leukocyte karyotyping

21   A 70-year-old woman was admitted with general weakness and lethargy. She was conscious and alert. Laboratory studies show Na⁺ of 122 mmol/l and urine osmolality of 650 mosmol/kg. The most appropriate initial therapy is

    ☐   **A**   Fluid restriction
    ☐   **B**   Demeclocycline therapy
    ☐   **C**   Hypertonic saline
    ☐   **D**   Lithium therapy
    ☐   **E**   Isotonic saline

22   A 60-year-old man was referred for further assessment. His wife has noticed that he is vague and distant. She also stated that he is unable to sleep and more recently has recurrent bouts of acute confusion. Which of the following is most suggestive of an organic delirium rather than a psychiatric disease?

    ☐   **A**   Confusion with regard to personal identity, time and place
    ☐   **B**   Normal ability to calculate
    ☐   **C**   Auditory hallucinations
    ☐   **D**   Normal electroencephalogram
    ☐   **E**   Positive Babinski sign

23   A 35-year-old man was referred because of enlarged breasts. On examination the breasts were large and firm fibrous tissue of more than 4 cm diameter was palpable within the breast tissue on both sides. Each of the following clinical situations could be responsible for this condition, except

    ☐   **A**   Carcinoma of the bronchus
    ☐   **B**   Spironolactone therapy
    ☐   **C**   Hyperthyroidism
    ☐   **D**   Enalapril therapy
    ☐   **E**   Testicular tumour

24 A 35-year-old man is admitted to the Emergency Department because of sudden severe pain and swelling in the right knee. He is unable to weight-bear and is shivering early in the morning. Examination of the knee reveals a hot, red and very tender knee. There was evidence of fluid collection in the knee. Neither passive nor active movement is possible. Some 20 ml of cloudy synovial fluid is aspirated and sent for Gram stain and culture. The organism most likely to be isolated is

☐ A *Neisseria gonorrhoeae*
☐ B *Chlamydia trachomatis*
☐ C *Staphylococcus aureus*
☐ D *Streptococcus pneumoniae*
☐ E *Staphylococcus epidermidis*

25 A 25-year-old obese woman has round facies, mental retardation and short fourth and fifth metacarpal bones. Laboratory studies show: Ca^{2+} 1.6 mmol/l, raised phosphate and PTH levels. The most likely diagnosis is

☐ A Cushing's syndrome
☐ B Osteoporosis
☐ C Primary hyperparathyroidism
☐ D Pseudohypoparathyroidism
☐ E Multiple endocrine neoplasia syndrome (MEN I)

26 A 30-year-old man with insulin-dependent diabetes and hypothyroidism develops fatigue, weight loss, and increasing pigmentation of the skin and buccal mucosa. The most likely cause of the recent complaint is

☐ A Vitiligo
☐ B Panhypopituitarism
☐ C Addison's disease
☐ D Coeliac disease
☐ E Peutz–Jeghers syndrome

27 A 58-year-old woman is admitted with sudden onset of weakness and loss of sensation of the right upper arm and right face. Further assessment revealed receptive and expressive dysphasia. The artery most likely to be involved in this stroke syndrome is

- [ ] **A** Basilar artery
- [ ] **B** Right vertebral artery
- [ ] **C** Left middle cerebral artery
- [ ] **D** Left anterior cerebral artery
- [ ] **E** Left posterior cerebral artery

28 A 50-year-old woman with dry mouth and dry eyes has arthritis affecting the knees and elbows. She was found to have positive Schirmer's test and is positive for anti-Ro antibodies. Each of the following disorders may be associated with this disease except

- [ ] **A** Lymphoma
- [ ] **B** Renal tubular acidosis
- [ ] **C** Primary biliary cirrhosis
- [ ] **D** Hypothyroidism
- [ ] **E** Sarcoidosis

29 A 20-year-old woman presents with sudden onset of swelling of the lips and tongue. She also has abdominal pain and vomiting. Her mother confirmed that her daughter had similar attacks over the years and even as a child. A brother and older sister have the same disorder. Which of the following statements about this disease is accurate?

- [ ] **A** It has sex-linked inheritance
- [ ] **B** Animal allergen is often identified in the house
- [ ] **C** Serum C4 is low
- [ ] **D** Antinuclear antibodies (ANA) are often positive
- [ ] **E** Raised IgE helps differentiate it from other immune disorders

30 A 15-year-old boy presented with arthralgia, skin rash and haematuria. Renal biopsy showed focal necrotising glomerulonephritis with diffuse mesangial IgA deposits. The most likely diagnosis is

☐ A Systemic lupus erythematosus (SLE)
☐ B Henoch–Schönlein purpura
☐ C Juvenile rheumatoid arthritis
☐ D Post-streptococcal glomerulonephritis
☐ E Goodpasture's syndrome

31 A 40-year-old chronic alcoholic is admitted with lassitude and lethargy. He reports numbness in the hands and around the mouth. Laboratory studies show normal renal function. The bone profile shows low Ca^{2+} (1.4 mmol/l) and raised phosphorus (1.8 mmol/l). The serum albumin was normal and the ALT was raised at 78 mmol/l. The most likely cause of the hypocalcaemia is

☐ A False reading (the corrected calcium is normal)
☐ B Hypomagnesaemia
☐ C Osteoporosis
☐ D Poor dietary intake of calcium
☐ E Intestinal malabsorption

32 A 72-year-old man has increasing difficulty with balance and frequent falls. He has an unblinking gaze and a monotonous voice. Which of the following signs is not indicative of Parkinson's disease?

☐ A Action tremor
☐ B Cogwheel rigidity
☐ C Bradykinesia
☐ D Micrographia
☐ E Loss of postural reflexes

33 A 45-year-old man is referred for further investigations. He has felt generally unwell with excessive tiredness and lethargy. He has noticed multiple bruises on the trunk and limbs. His blood test confirmed a prolonged bleeding time. Each of the following disorders could be responsible for this patient's presentation, except

☐ A Hereditary haemorrhagic telangiectasia (HHT)
☐ B Uraemia
☐ C Platelet storage-pool disease
☐ D Idiopathic thrombocytopenic purpura (ITP)
☐ E Essential thrombocytosis

34 A 55-year-old woman reports increasing fatigue and recent unsteady gait with a tendency to fall when she closes her eyes. The full blood count reveals a haemoglobin of 7 g/dl, MCV 112 fl and hypersegmented neutrophils. Which of the following is not a recognised neurological complication of this disorder?

☐ A Optic atrophy
☐ B Loss of sensation of smell
☐ C Impaired cognitive function
☐ D Grand mal seizure
☐ E Bilateral Babinski sign

35 A 56-year-old woman is referred for further assessment of chronic obstructive pulmonary disease. Each of the following clinical features is suggestive of potential reversibility of airflow obstruction, except

☐ A History of eczema
☐ B PaO_2 of 8 kPa
☐ C Nasal polyp
☐ D Normal pulmonary diffusion capacity
☐ E High peripheral blood eosinophil count

36 A 56-year-old woman reports progressive weakness in the lower limbs. Three months earlier she complained of sudden spontaneous backache which soon became persistent and disabling. Radiographs of the spine showed destruction of L1–L4 vertebrae. Which of the following is included among signs of a lower motor neurone lesion?

☐ **A** Muscle atrophy
☐ **B** Ankle clonus
☐ **C** Absent abdominal reflexes
☐ **D** Hyper-reflexia
☐ **E** Bilateral Babinski sign

37 A 60-year-old woman is noted to have a small pupil which is non-reactive to light but constricts to accommodation. The most likely cause for the pupil abnormality is

☐ **A** Holmes–Adie pupil
☐ **B** Posterior communicating artery syndrome
☐ **C** Pancoast's tumour
☐ **D** Syphilis
☐ **E** Pontine haemorrhage

38 A 31-year-old woman is referred because of unsteady gait and rigidity. Her problem started seven years ago with tremor affecting the arms and the head, associated with dysarthria and dysphagia. It is noted that she has deranged liver function tests and recently was referred to the ophthalmologist for an eye problem. The most likely diagnosis is

☐ **A** Huntington's disease
☐ **B** Multiple sclerosis
☐ **C** Ataxia telangiectasia
☐ **D** Wilson's disease
☐ **E** Parkinson's disease

39 A 30-year-old man who is known to have AIDS is referred because of an erythematous scaly eruption covering the cheeks and the forehead. The most likely diagnosis is

- ☐ **A** Rosacea
- ☐ **B** Discoid lupus
- ☐ **C** Psoriasis
- ☐ **D** Seborrhoeic dermatitis
- ☐ **E** Acne

40 A 60-year-old man complains of tiredness and lack of energy. His full blood count reveals: haemoglobin 7.9 g/dl, MCV 66 fl, platelet count 600 × 10⁹/l. The serum urea was elevated and the iron and ferritin levels were low. Which of the following statements about this condition is true?

- ☐ **A** A normal ferritin level excludes the diagnosis
- ☐ **B** Splenomegaly occurs in 20% of cases
- ☐ **C** The most probable cause of anaemia in this man is reduced iron intake
- ☐ **D** Iron stores in the bone marrow are usually well preserved, even in severe cases
- ☑ **E** The associated thrombocytosis is an indication of an underlying myeloproliferative disorder

41 A 50-year-old woman is admitted with high fever and a generalised headache. Examination reveals chemosis and cyanosis of the upper face. There was proptosis and ophthalmoplegia of the left eye. Pin prick sensation was lost from the left forehead. The most likely diagnosis is

- ☐ **A** Periorbital cellulitis
- ☐ **B** Osteomyelitis of the left maxillary sinus
- ☑ **C** Left retro-orbital tumour
- ☐ **D** Cavernous sinus thrombosis
- ☐ **E** Superior sagittal sinus thrombosis

42 A 61-year-old man has a long history of excessive bleeding which occurs following tooth extraction and other invasive procedures. He has learnt to avoid all competitive sports. The screening tests for haemostasis were all normal, including prothrombin time (PT), activated partial thromboplastin time (APTT), platelet count and bleeding time. Which of the following disorders is the most likely diagnosis?

☐ **A** Factor XIII deficiency
☐ **B** von Willebrand's disease
☐ **C** Haemophilia A
☐ **D** Factor C deficiency
☐ **E** Haemophilia B

43 A 41-year-old man was admitted to the Emergency Department with skin rash, rigors and temperature spike of 39.9°C. The full blood count revealed a WBC of 2.3×10^9/l and neutrophil count of 0.5×10^9/l. Each of the following statements about this blood abnormality is true, except

☐ **A** Vitamin B_{12} and folic acid levels should be obtained
☐ **B** If carbimazole is the offending agent on this occasion, future use of the drug is contraindicated
☐ **C** Perianal abscess is a common presenting symptom
☐ **D** Difficulty in swallowing may be due to associated *Candida* infection
☐ **E** Chickenpox might rapidly progress to severe and fatal haemorrhagic varicella

44 A 61-year-old man is admitted because of increasing confusion and inadequately controlled lower backache. He is found to have multiple myeloma. Which of the following statements regarding this patient's disease is correct?

☐ **A** Osteoporotic vertebral collapse fracture may be responsible for his backache
☐ **B** Radiotherapy is ineffective in treating bone pain
☐ **C** Isotope bone scanning is more sensitive for identifying early disease
☐ **D** Plain radiographs of the spine would show typical widespread osteoblastic bone lesions
☐ **E** The hypercalcaemia is usually steroid-resistant

45 An 88-year-old woman is referred because of a tense bullous eruption on the inner sides of the upper and lower limbs as well as the abdomen. The most likely diagnosis is

  ☐ **A** Pemphigus
  ☑ **B** Bullous pemphigoid
  ☐ **C** Herpes zoster
  ☐ **D** Dermatitis herpetiformis
  ☐ **E** Stevens-Johnson syndrome

46 A teacher has brought his son to you because he is very worried that his son might be suffering with haemophilia. Which one of the following best excludes a diagnosis of haemophilia?

  ☐ **A** Normal activated partial thromboplastin time
  ☐ **B** Normal prothrombin time
  ☐ **C** Absence of excessive bleeding after tooth extraction
  ☐ **D** Absence of spontaneous bleeding episodes
  ☐ **E** Absence of family history

47 A 64-year-old builder who had a surgical operation for inguinal hernia a develops a wound infection a week later and methicillin-resistant *Staphylococcus aureus* (MRSA) is recovered from the wound. Which one of the following isolation techniques do you think is appropriate in this condition?

  ☐ **A** Enteric precautions
  ☐ **B** Blood and body fluid precautions
  ☐ **C** Respiratory isolation only
  ☐ **D** Strict isolation
  ☑ **E** Contact isolation

48 A 40-year-old male dancer presents with thrombophlebitis of the lower limb. Examination reveals five painless, punched-out ulcers on the scrotum with concomitant oral ulcers. Which of the following is the most likely diagnosis?

☐ **A** Granuloma inguinale
☐ **B** Syphilis
☐ **C** Herpes simplex genitalis
☐ **D** Behçet's disease
☐ **E** Systemic lupus erythematosus

49 A 20-year-old car mechanic who has been abusing inhalants for many years was admitted with sudden collapse. The ambulance crew said he was inhaling solvent by rebreathing from a plastic bag. He is transferred to the Intensive Care Unit. A few minutes later he stops breathing and the cardiac monitor records ventricular fibrillation rhythm. In resuscitating this patient which one of the following should be avoided?

☐ **A** Direct current shock
☐ **B** Intubation
☐ **C** Oxygen therapy
☐ **D** Intravenous β-blocker
☐ **E** Intravenous adrenaline (epinephrine)

50 Patients admitted to a hospital with confirmed diagnosis of acute appendicitis were audited over a six-month period. The mean length of hospital stay was 9 days, SD = 7 days and median = 5 days. Which one of the following is the most accurate statement about length of hospital stay for these patients?

☐ **A** Half of the patients stayed 9 days or longer
☐ **B** Length of stay follows a negatively skewed distribution
☐ **C** The range of length of stay was 14 days
☐ **D** More than 50% of patients stayed 4 days or more
☐ **E** About 2.5% of patients had a length of stay above 23 days

51 A 24-year-old male inpatient appears confused and is behaving in an unusual manner on the ward. Nursing staff report a disrupted sleep pattern. The patient has no psychiatric history. You wish to exclude an organic cause for his behaviour and order an electroencephalogram (EEG). In which of the following disorders are EEG abnormalities least expected?

- [ ] A Herpes simplex encephalitis
- [ ] B Interictal psychosis
- [ ] C Metabolic encephalopathy
- [ ] D Hebephrenic schizophrenia
- [ ] E Subacute sclerosing panencephalitis

52 A 62-year-old man presented with several non-healing ulcerated lesions on the lower extremities and hand, present for approximately three years. He relates that each lesion began as a tender erythematous papule that subsequently ulcerated. The lesions have failed to respond to topical steroids and topical antifungal agents. He received skin grafts over the lower extremity lesions one year ago but the grafts ulcerated. There are multiple ulcerated lesions bilaterally on the lower extremities and one on the right hand. The lesions have dusky purple margins and a halo of erythema. They range in size from 2.5 to 6 cm in diameter. The bases of the ulcers are verrucous with regions of necrosis and granulation tissue. The most likely diagnosis is

- [ ] A Venous insufficiency
- [ ] B Pyoderma gangrenosum
- [ ] C Tropical ulcer
- [ ] D Bacterial skin infection
- [ ] E Ischaemic ulcers

53 A 58-year-old chronic alcoholic was admitted with increasing shortness of breath and a distended abdomen. Physical examination revealed evidence for ascites and pitting oedema in both legs. The pulse was 94 bpm, blood pressure 110/60 mmHg and the jugular venous pressure was not raised. The condition least likely to be responsible for this clinical presentation is

- [ ] **A** Alcoholic cardiomyopathy
- [ ] **B** Liver cirrhosis
- [ ] **C** Bowel cancer with liver metastasis
- [ ] **D** Tuberculous peritonitis
- [ ] **E** Portal vein thrombosis

54 A 40-year-old Egyptian tourist is admitted with haematemesis. He is known to have chronic liver disease caused by *Schistosoma mansoni* infection. Physical examination would reveal which one of the following clinical signs?

- [ ] **A** Splenomegaly
- [ ] **B** Jaundice
- [ ] **C** Ascites
- [ ] **D** Spider nevi
- [ ] **E** Gynaecomastia

55 A 35-year-old healthy man was seen for an annual medical review as part of his company employment policy. Examination reveals oral thrush in an otherwise fit and healthy man. Further tests confirm oral candidiasis. He denies any illness and he is receiving no drugs. Which one of the following is the most likely underlying disease?

- [ ] **A** Lymphoma
- [ ] **B** Alcoholism
- [ ] **C** HIV infection
- [ ] **D** Chronic renal failure
- [ ] **E** Heroin addiction

56 A 72-year-old woman is admitted to the Coronary Care Unit with an acute inferior myocardial infarction. During ECG recording it is noticed that her heart rate is 40 bpm with sinus rhythm and blood pressure is 87/55 mmHg. The most appropriate immediate action is

- [ ] **A** Keep monitoring the pulse and the blood pressure for a further 24 hours
- [ ] **B** Insert temporary pacemaker
- [ ] **C** Organise emergency percutaneous coronary angioplasty
- [ ] **D** Give 24-hour isoprenaline infusion
- [ ] **E** Give intravenous atropine sulphate (0.6 mg)

57 An 80-year-old man is referred from a nursing home with fever, rigors, nausea and vomiting. He is bedridden and has sacral decubitus ulcers. Blood cultures grow *Streptococcus milleri*. The most likely site of infection is?

- [ ] **A** Sacral bedsores
- [ ] **B** Urinary tract infection
- [ ] **C** Liver abscess
- [ ] **D** Endocarditis
- [ ] **E** Osteomyelitis

58 A 50-year-old accountant is referred for investigation of fever and general ill health. His initial renal function tests show: urea 45 mmol/l, creatinine 480 μmol/l. Which one of the following medication dose interval should be most prolonged when used in this patient?

- [ ] **A** Gentamicin
- [ ] **B** Amoxicillin
- [ ] **C** Vancomycin
- [ ] **D** Penicillin
- [ ] **E** Cefuroxime

59 A 38-year-old woman presents with bilateral pitting ankle oedema. The jugular venous pressure is not raised and the hepatojugular reflux was negative. The woman's ankle oedema would not be explained by which of the following conditions?

☐ **A** Pelvic tumour
☐ **B** Amlodipine therapy
☐ **C** Cyclic oedema
☐ **D** Hypoalbuminaemia
☐ **E** Right heart failure

60 A 68-year-old man presents with recent onset headache and vomiting. Ophthalmoscopy reveals optic atrophy in the right eye and papilloedema in the left one. The most likely diagnosis is?

☐ **A** Pinealoma
☐ **B** Medulloblastoma
☐ **C** Acoustic neuroma
☐ **D** Sphenoid wing meningioma
☐ **E** Pituitary adenoma

61 An 85-year-old man is referred with a three-month history of dysphagia. Barium swallow showed a filling defect in the oesophagus. Gastro-oesophagoscopy and biopsy confirmed the presence of squamous cell carcinoma of the oesophagus. Each of the following conditions might be associated with this tumour, except

☐ **A** Achalasia
☐ **B** Smoking
☐ **C** Tylosis
☐ **D** Barrett's oesophagus
☐ **E** Head and neck cancer

62 A 50-year-old publican is referred with anuria. The initial renal function test showed the urea at 45 mmol/l and the creatinine at 480 μmol/l. A urine sample from a catheter was strongly positive for myoglobin. This clinical picture can develop as a result of each of the following clinical situations except

☐ **A** Alcohol ingestion
☐ **B** Hypokalaemia
☐ **C** Barbiturate overdose
☐ **D** Hypophosphataemia
☐ **E** Hypocalcaemia

63 A 40-year-old man has a six-month history of increasing shortness of breath and wheeze. The full blood count shows an increased absolute eosinophil count. Chest X-ray and a CT scan of the chest show right apical bronchiectasis. Which one of the following is the most likely diagnosis?

☐ **A** Loeffler's syndrome
☐ **B** Allergic bronchopulmonary aspergillosis
☐ **C** Polyarteritis nodosa
☐ **D** Nitrofurantoin hypersensitivity
☐ **E** *Strongyloides stercoralis* infection

64 A 56-year-old man is referred with dyspnoea and cough productive of putrid green sputum of four weeks duration. The chest X-ray shows cavity formation in the left lower lobe. He has advanced motor neurone disease. This clinical picture is most likely to be caused by infection with

☐ **A** *Legionella pneumophila*
☐ **B** *Mycoplasma pneumoniae*
☐ **C** *Streptococcus pneumoniae*
☐ **D** Anaerobic bacteria
☐ **E** Common cold virus

65 A 75-year-old woman is admitted with left lower lobe pneumonia. She was given a course of cephalosporin antibiotics and she improved. However, at the end of the course she started to have diarrhoea, passing a watery stool. Investigations confirmed the diagnosis of pseudomembranous colitis. Each of the following oral medications is beneficial in treating this condition, except

☐ **A** Vancomycin
☐ **B** Bacitracin
☐ **C** Colestyramine
☐ **D** Flagyl®
☐ **E** Gentamicin

66 A 38-year-old woman has dyspnoea on exertion and orthopnoea. Examination reveals a loud first heart sound, a diastolic rumble, and a large *v* wave in the jugular pulse. The most likely diagnosis is

☐ **A** Mitral stenosis and tricuspid regurgitation
☐ **B** Isolated mitral stenosis
☐ **C** Aortic regurgitation
☐ **D** Mitral regurgitation and tricuspid regurgitation
☐ **E** Tricuspid regurgitation

67 A 35-year old woman has slurred speech and a progressive gait disturbance. Magnetic resonance imaging (MRI) shows several focal abnormalities in the periventricular areas, normal sized ventricles and no space occupying lesion. The cerebellum was also normal. The most likely diagnosis is

☐ **A** Motor neurone disease
☐ **B** Friedreich's ataxia
☐ **C** Multiple sclerosis (MS)
☐ **D** Syphilis
☐ **E** Huntington's disease

68 A 22-year-old woman has a three-month history of fatigue of insidious onset, poor appetite and athralgia. She has no previous history of liver disease. She takes thyroxine replacement therapy. Physical examination reveals spider naevi and hepatomegaly. The ALT is five-times higher than the normal. Her disease is most likely be associated with

☐ A Antimitochondrial antibodies
☐ B Low serum caeruloplasmin levels
☐ C Anti-parietal cell antibodies
☐ D Anti-smooth muscle antibodies
☐ E Hepatitis B surface antigen (HbsAg)

69 A 65-year-old obese man presents with recurrent episodes of cough. His wife said his coughing attacks disturb her sleep almost every night. He noticed that his voice is hoarse in the morning. He has never smoked and has no history of cardiac or respiratory problems. There is no history of allergy and the chest X-ray is normal. The procedure most likely to yield crucial diagnostic information is

☐ A Pulmonary function tests
☐ B 24-hour pH monitoring of the lower oesophagus
☐ C High-resolution CT scan of the chest
☐ D Barium swallow
☐ E Indirect laryngoscopy

70 A 38-year-old man has a six-month history of diarrhoea, abdominal pain and tenesmus. Flexible sigmoidoscopy reveals proctitis. A biopsy specimen shows acute and chronic inflammation. Each of the following statements is true about this disorder, except

☐ A There is an increased risk of gastrointestinal malignancy
☐ B Other family members are likely to develop the same illness
☐ C Steatorrhoea is likely to develop as a result of pancreatic insufficiency
☐ D The likelihood of renal stones will increase
☐ E The likelihood of gallstones will increase

71 A 38-year-old man has a six-month history of insidious onset of fatigue, poor appetite and jaundice. The serum aspartate aminotransferase (AST) to alanine aminotransferase (ALT) ratio is greater than 2:1. Ultrasound examination of the liver shows no evidence of cirrhosis. The most likely diagnosis is

☐ **A** Viral hepatitis
☐ **B** Alcoholic hepatitis
☐ **C** Cholangitis
☐ **D** Autoimmune hepatitis
☐ **E** Haemolytic anaemia

72 A 68-year-old woman presents with a six-month history of insidious onset of fatigue, poor appetite and morning stiffness predominantly in the shoulders. Physical examination was unremarkable except for pallor. Laboratory studies reveal normal WBC, haematocrit of 27%, MCV 70 fl, platelets 700 × 10^9/l and ESR 78 mm/h. Bone marrow aspirate is normal, with increased iron stores. The most likely diagnosis is

☐ **A** Essential thrombocytosis
☐ **B** Hypothyroidism
☐ **C** Myelodysplasia
☐ **D** Polymyalgia rheumatica
☐ **E** Polycythaemia rubra vera

73 A 28-year-old woman presents with extreme pallor, palpitations and lack of energy. The full blood count reveals: haemoglobin 4 g/dl, WBC 12 × 10^9/l, MCV 112 fl, platelet count of 500 × 10^9/l, reticulocyte count 20%. The finding of depleted iron stores is highly suggestive of which of the following conditions?

☐ **A** Sickle cell anaemia
☐ **B** Thalassaemia major
☐ **C** IgG warm antibody mediated haemolytic anaemia
☐ **D** Spherocytosis
☐ **E** Paroxysmal nocturnal haemoglobinuria

74 A 30-year-old woman is referred because of recent onset headache and dizziness. Physical examination reveals blue lips and blue fingertips. Urgent blood gases on air show a Pao_2 of 12 kPa. This patient is probably taking which one of the following medications?

- ☐ **A** Dapsone
- ☐ **B** Sodium valproate
- ☐ **C** Phenytoin
- ☐ **D** Zinc sulphate
- ☐ **E** Nitrous oxide

75 A 40-year-old man has epistaxis and bruises easily. As a child he had excessive bleeding following tonsillectomy and teeth extractions. His mother and sister had similar symptoms. The most likely diagnosis is?

- ☐ **A** Haemophilia A
- ☐ **B** Haemophilia B
- ☐ **C** von Willebrand's disease
- ☐ **D** Idiopathic thrombocytopenic purpura
- ☐ **E** Lupus anticoagulant

76 A 22-year-old man with haemophilia A has plasma factor VIII levels of less than 1%. Spontaneous bleeding would most likely manifest as

- ☐ **A** Haemarthrosis
- ☐ **B** Petechial haemorrhages around the ankles
- ☐ **C** Haematuria
- ☐ **D** Cerebral haemorrhage
- ☐ **E** Haematemesis

77 A 40-year-old engineer who has smoked a pack of cigarettes daily for 20 years presents with chronic unproductive cough associated with a history of recurrent pneumothoraces and chronic hepatitis. The most likely diagnosis is

☐ **A** Marfan's syndrome
☐ **B** Cystic fibrosis
☐ **C** Immotile cilia syndrome
☐ **D** α_1-Antitrypsin deficiency
☐ **E** Chronic bronchitis

78 A 38-year-old man was referred with a palpable mass in the left upper quadrant of the abdomen. This finding is consistent with each of the following conditions, except

☐ **A** Hereditary spherocytosis
☐ **B** Chronic myeloid leukaemia
☐ **C** Polycythaemia rubra vera
☐ **D** Sickle cell disease
☐ **E** β-Thalassaemia

79 A 34-year-old man presents with a three-week history of a rash on his abdomen and trunk. He first noticed a red, slightly pruritic lesion just to the left of his umbilicus several weeks ago. It was scaly and slightly raised. About seven days later several similar but smaller lesions began to appear around the initial one. They continued to spread until they covered his entire abdomen and chest. On examination there is a 3 cm × 1 cm oval lesion lateral to his umbilicus. It is erythematous, scaly and dry-appearing, with surrounding excoriations. The other lesions on his trunk appear the same except they are smaller. The most likely diagnosis is

☐ **A** Tinea versicolor
☐ **B** Guttate psoriasis
☐ **C** Drug eruption
☐ **D** Pityriasis rosea
☐ **E** Secondary syphilis

80 You are asked to review a 38-year-old man whose peripheral blood picture shows fragmented erythrocytes (schistocytes). This finding is characteristic of each of the following disorders, except

☐ **A** Disseminated intravascular coagulation (DIC)
☐ **B** Liver cirrhosis
☐ **C** Malignant hypertension
☐ **D** Prosthetic heart valve trauma
☐ **E** Thrombotic thrombocytopenic purpura

81 A 38-year-old woman was brought to the Emergency Department because of headache, difficulty in concentrating and slurred speech. She had previously been in excellent health. She was found to have fever, anaemia (haemoglobin 8.4 g/dl) and profound thrombocytopenia, platelets 30 × 10⁹/l, 20 × 10⁹/l (normal range 150–400 × 10⁹/l). Schistocytes were present on the peripheral blood film and the serum lactate dehydrogenase (LDH) level was five times above the normal limits. The most likely diagnosis is

☐ **A** Idiopathic thrombocytopenic purpura (ITP)
☐ **B** Thalassaemia major
☐ **C** Thrombotic thrombocytopenic purpura (TTP)
☐ **D** Autoimmune haemolytic anaemia
☐ **E** Aplastic anaemia

82 A 46-year-old dentist was referred for investigation of dark brown-coloured urine. He was found to have anaemia (haemoglobin 8.4 g/dl), leukopenia, thrombocytopenia and an elevated reticulocyte count. The serum LDH level was five times above the normal limits. Which of the following laboratory tests is most helpful in identifying this disorder?

☐ **A** Acid haemolysis test
☐ **B** Bone marrow aspiration
☐ **C** Coombs' test
☐ **D** Red cell mass
☐ **E** Urine haemoglobin

83 A 68-year-old woman with carcinoma of the bronchus with bone metastases has a one-week history of progressive lethargy, nausea and vomiting, constipation, polyuria and polydipsia. She has been taking morphine for three weeks. The most likely cause for the recent deterioration is

- ☐ **A** Adverse reaction to morphine
- ☐ **B** Large bowel obstruction
- ☐ **C** Brain metastases
- ☐ **D** Hypercalcaemia
- ☐ **E** Urinary tract infection

84 A 34-year-old man with haemophilia came to you asking for further clarification about the chances of his children acquiring the same disease. He has four sons and four daughters. His wife's family has no history of haemophilia. Which one of the following statements is true?

- ☐ **A** All the sons will be normal
- ☐ **B** All the sons will be carriers
- ☐ **C** Half the sons will be affected
- ☐ **D** Half the daughters will be carriers
- ☐ **E** Half the daughters will be affected

85 A 78-year-old man is brought to his General Practitioner by his wife. She reports an 18-month history of progressive impairment in memory (especially for recent events), worsening apathy and occasional disorientation in previously familiar environments. He scores 21/30 on the Mini Mental State examination. BP is 150/90 mmHg, pulse 80 bpm (regular). Which one of the following is the most likely diagnosis?

- ☐ **A** Alzheimer's disease
- ☐ **B** Depression
- ☐ **C** Mild cognitive impairment
- ☐ **D** Lewy Body dementia
- ☐ **E** Vascular dementia

86　An otherwise healthy but morbidly obese non-smoking 43-year-old man is referred as part of a preliminary assessment for a weight reduction programme. He is likely to have a significant reduction in all of the following, except

   ☐　A　Forced expiratory volume in 1 second (FEV_1)
   ☐　B　Forced vital capacity (FVC)
   ☐　C　Functional residual capacity (FRC)
   ☐　D　Diffusing capacity for carbon monoxide (DLCO)
   ☐　E　Expiratory reserve volume (ERV)

87　Three days after a chest infection a 20-year-old insulin-dependent diabetic starts to have nausea, abdominal pain and vomiting. The blood glucose was 24 mmol/l and arterial blood pH was 7.25. Which one of the following abnormal blood results is rarely encountered in this condition?

   ☐　A　Hyperkalaemia
   ☐　B　A rise in plasma chloride
   ☐　C　A low $Paco_2$
   ☐　D　Tetany
   ☐　E　A low bicarbonate

88　Two months after undergoing a right mastectomy for carcinoma of the breast a 50-year-old patient is scheduled for radiotherapy to eliminate the remaining malignant cells. The most sensitive structure in a cell to radiotherapy is

   ☐　A　Cell membrane
   ☐　B　Mitochondrial membrane
   ☐　C　DNA
   ☐　D　Plasma membrane
   ☐　E　Cell enzymes

89 A 20-year-old man from Africa was investigated for anaemia. Haemoglobin electrophoresis shows increased Hb A$_2$ levels. This abnormality is most often encountered in which of the following types of anaemia?

☐ **A** Hereditary spherocytosis
☐ **B** Sideroblastic anaemia
☐ **C** β-Thalassaemia
☐ **D** Iron deficiency anaemia
☐ **E** α-Thalassaemia

90 A 30-year-old man is admitted with sore throat and cervical lymphadenopathy. Epstein–Barr virus (EBV) antigens are identified. Each of the following diseases are caused by EBV infection except

☐ **A** Burkitt's lymphoma
☐ **B** Infectious mononucleosis
☐ **C** Kaposi's sarcoma
☐ **D** Oral hairy leukoplakia
☐ **E** Nasopharyngeal carcinoma

91 A routine annual health check on a bank employee shows raised serum bilirubin levels. Bilirubin is derived from each of the following, except

☐ **A** Haemoglobin
☐ **B** Cholesterol
☐ **C** Catalase
☐ **D** Myoglobin
☐ **E** Cytochromes

92 A 31-year-old woman presented with dysuria and frequency of micturition. Urine microscopy shows a high number of white cells but no organisms are detected. Urine cultures are negative. The clinical picture is typical of each of the following disorders, except

   ☐ **A** Renal tuberculosis
   ☐ **B** *Escherichia coli* infection
   ☐ **C** *Ureaplasma urealyticum* infection
   ☐ **D** Candidiasis
   ☐ **E** Urolithiasis

93 A 24-year-old woman has a webbed neck, short stature amenorrhoea and 45 chromosomes. The most likely associated cardiac malformation in this condition is

   ☐ **A** Atrial septal defect
   ☐ **B** Patent ductus arteriosus
   ☐ **C** Ventricular septal defect
   ☐ **D** Pulmonary stenosis
   ☐ **E** Coarctation of the aorta

94 A course of treatment with an alkylating agent is planned after initial steroid therapy for a 60-year-old man with fibrosing alveolitis. Alkylating agents are a group of cytotoxic drugs that includes each of the following, except

   ☐ **A** Melphalan
   ☐ **B** Chlorambucil
   ☐ **C** Vincristine
   ☐ **D** Nitrogen mustard
   ☐ **E** Busulfan

95 Adding an angiotensin-converting enzyme inhibitor (ACEI) is considered the next appropriate step in treating a 56-year-old man with hypertension who is poorly controlled on bendroflumethiazide (bendrofluazide) and β-blockers. ACEIs are effective because they inhibit the actions of angiotensin II, which include each of the following, except

☐ A Peripheral vasoconstriction
☐ B Stimulation of thirst
☐ C Stimulation of aldosterone secretion
☐ D Inhibition of ADH secretion
☐ E Stimulation of cardiac hypertrophy

96 A 30-year-old man investigated for excessive sweating was found to have a mass in the right adrenal gland. Hormones exclusively secreted by the adrenal medulla include

☐ A Adrenaline (epinephrine)
☐ B Androgen
☐ C Aldosterone
☐ D Antidiuretic hormone
☐ E Cortisol

97 A 50-year-old man is referred by his doctor with double vision. The patient was well until early this morning. His doctor suggests paralysis of the third cranial nerve as the cause of the diplopia. A palsy of the third cranial nerve will result in which apparent direction of gaze of the affected eyeball?

☐ A Medial
☐ B Superolateral
☐ C Superomedial
☐ D Inferolateral
☐ E Inferomedial

98 A 30-year-old man was found to have hypertension. Which one of the following statements about evaluating patients for secondary hypertension is correct?

☐ A About 75% of patients with renovascular hypertension have an abdominal bruit

☐ B Diastolic hypertension and muscle weakness are often present in patients with hyperthyroidism

☐ C Assessing growth hormone level is helpful in diagnosing hyperparathyroidism

☐ D Computed tomography of the adrenals is the initial step for diagnosing suspected phaeochromocytoma

☐ E Patients suspected of having Cushing's syndrome should undergo a dexamethasone suppression test

99 A 30-year-old woman presented with a six-month history of loose bowel motions and weight loss. Which one of the following is the gold standard test for the diagnosis of gluten-sensitive enteropathy?

☐ A Constellation of compatible symptoms
☐ B Elevated IgA anti-endomysial antibody levels
☐ C Small bowel biopsy
☐ D Presence of IgA antibodies to gliadin
☐ E Presence of IgG antibodies to gliadin

100 A 23-year-old trainee nurse presents with anxiety about needles. This has developed to the extent that she is very anxious and distressed when in the treatment room with sealed packs of needles and finds it impossible to handle a sheathed needle. Her symptoms are beginning to affect her training. Select the most appropriate initial treatment approach for this patient.

☐ A Paroxetine
☐ B Psychoanalytic psychotherapy
☐ C Risperidone
☐ D Relaxation therapy
☐ E Cognitive behavioural therapy

PAPER TWO QUESTIONS

101 A 20-year-old man is rushed in to the Emergency Department drowsy and confused. The ambulance crew state that he has swallowed an unknown quantity of antifreeze liquid. Which one of the following clinical or laboratory findings is not suggestive of antifreeze liquid ingestion?

- [ ] **A** Pulmonary oedema
- [ ] **B** Metabolic alkalosis
- [ ] **C** An elevated anion gap
- [ ] **D** A decreased level of consciousness
- [ ] **E** Urinary calcium oxalate crystals

102 You have been called to review a 66-year-old lawyer who presents with weakness in the limbs. The CT scan of the brain shows a temporal lobe tumour. Each of the following clinical features are typical of a lesion in this area, except

- [ ] **A** Homonymous hemianopia
- [ ] **B** Visual hallucinations
- [ ] **C** *Déjà vu*
- [ ] **D** Receptive dysphasia
- [ ] **E** Ataxic nystagmus

103 A 30-year-old nurse has diarrhoea-predominant irritable bowel syndrome (IBS). She has tried herbal medicine in the past. In your opinion which one of the following agents is she most likely to respond to?

- [ ] **A** Smooth-muscle relaxants
- [ ] **B** Antispasmodic agents
- [ ] **C** Amitriptyline
- [ ] **D** Prednisone enema
- [ ] **E** Loperamide

104 A 60-year-old woman developed sudden loss of vision in the left eye. She saw her doctor immediately who arranged a few tests and organised referral to the eye specialist. Two days later she suddenly loses vision in the second eye. Which one of the following is the most likely cause of the blindness?

- ☐ **A** Papilloedema
- ☑ **B** Giant cell arteritis
- ☐ **C** Open angle glaucoma
- ☐ **D** Migraine vasospasm
- ☐ **E** Retinal vein occlusion

105 A 58-year-old man with chronic obstructive pulmonary disease is admitted with an acute infective exacerbation. Two hours after admission he becomes stuporous and disorientated. You notice that he was given intravenous cephalosporin and was inhaling 60% oxygen through a face mask. The blood gases show: $PaCO_2$ 11 kPa, PaO_2 16 kPa. Each of the following therapeutic measures are appropriate at this stage, except

- ☐ **A** Consider aminophylline infusion
- ☑ **B** Stop oxygen therapy immediately
- ☐ **C** Use nebulised bronchodilators
- ☐ **D** Give steroid therapy
- ☐ **E** Organise chest physiotherapy

106 A 17-year-old girl who takes the contraceptive pill has been diagnosed with epilepsy. She expresses her wishes to continue with the Pill as she is not planning to have children in the near future. Which one of the following would be the best choice of antiepileptic medication?

- ☐ **A** Topiramate
- ☐ **B** Carbamazepine
- ☐ **C** Phenytoin
- ☐ **D** Valproate
- ☐ **E** Barbiturate

107 A 40-year-old woman who is known to have had multiple sclerosis (MS) for three years presents with impaired visual acuity. Which one of the following would physical examination of the eyes most likely reveal?

☐ **A** Choroiditis
☐ **B** Optic neuritis
☐ **C** Internuclear ophthalmoplegia
☐ **D** Retinal detachment
☐ **E** Macular oedema

108 A 57-year-old woman with a 15-year history of rheumatoid arthritis (RA) is referred for further assessment. She was maintained on steroids after she failed trials with sulfasalazine and methotrexate, despite initial success with each drug. You decide to consider her for treatment with one of the biological agents. Blocking the biological function of which one of the following molecules will provide significant anti-inflammatory effect in RA?

☐ **A** Interleukin-10 (IL-10)
☐ **B** Interleukin-4 (IL-4)
☐ **C** Interleukin-1 (IL-1)
☐ **D** Soluble tumour necrosis factor (TNF) receptors
☐ **E** Transforming growth factor-beta (TGF-β)

109 A 66-year-old man presents with poor appetite and general malaise. Physical examination reveals palpable lymph nodes. The finding of lymph nodes in which one of the following areas is most likely to be suggestive of malignancy?

☐ **A** Cervical
☐ **B** Supraclavicular
☐ **C** Epitrochlear
☐ **D** Axillary
☐ **E** Inguinal

110 A 66-year-old man is referred for further investigation of an enlarged left supraclavicular lymph node. Which one of the following is the diagnostic technique of choice for evaluating lymphadenopathy if neoplasm is suspected?

- [ ] **A** Computed tomography (CT scan)
- [ ] **B** Magnetic resonance imaging (MRI)
- [ ] **C** Open biopsy
- [ ] **D** Fine-needle aspiration
- [ ] **E** Incisional wedge biopsy

111 A 60-year-old man with hypertension and diabetes presents with sudden loss of vision in the right eye. The retina was pale with a cherry-red spot at the macula. Which one of the following is the most likely diagnosis?

- [ ] **A** Diabetic retinopathy
- [ ] **B** Hypertensive retinopathy
- [ ] **C** Retinal artery occlusion
- [ ] **D** Retinal detachment
- [ ] **E** Retinal vein occlusion

112 You are called to see an abnormal 12-lead ECG recording from a 67-year-old man with atrial fibrillation who has been on digoxin for two years. He has hypokalaemia and you suspect digoxin toxicity. Which one of the following is the rhythm least likely to be related to digoxin toxicity?

- [ ] **A** First-degree heart block
- [ ] **B** Mobitz type I (Wenckebach)
- [ ] **C** Mobitz type II second-degree atrioventricular (AV) block
- [ ] **D** Third-degree (complete) heart block
- [ ] **E** AV junctional rhythms

113 A 23-year-old male dancer in a nightclub attends Casualty two days after an episode of prolonged retrosternal pain, accompanied by intense sweating, following cocaine use. During the examination, the patient is anxious and hyperactive. An electrocardiogram reveals acute ST elevation, T-wave inversion, and pathological Q waves. The cardiac enzymes (creatinine kinase and troponin T) were significantly elevated. He is admitted to the Coronary Care Unit. Which one of the following medications should be avoided at this stage?

☐ **A** Atenolol
☐ **B** Aspirin
☐ **C** Glyceryl trinitrate
☐ **D** Benzodiazepine
☐ **E** Verapamil

114 A 20-year-old man is referred because of abnormal behaviour. The initial manifestation of this was when he was responding to apparent auditory hallucinations, as if he believed he was Jesus Christ. He also placed food he had prepared for his brother in a dog-dish. More recently, he has become quite aggressive. He assaulted a friend with a rock, apparently laughing throughout and after the incident. With regard to the management of this patient, which one of the following statements is true?

☐ **A** Early combination therapy (of different antipsychotic medications) at the outset is the treatment of choice
☐ **B** Clozapine treatment should be monitored with fortnightly liver function tests
☐ **C** Electroconvulsive therapy (ECT) is effective treatment in certain patients with schizophrenia
☐ **D** Atypical antipsychotic drug use is not associated with increased risk of neuroleptic malignant syndrome
☐ **E** Antidepressants are generally contraindicated in schizophrenia

115 A 55-year-old mechanic presents with deranged liver function tests, diabetes mellitus and slate-grey hyperpigmentation of the skin. Hereditary haemochromatosis is confirmed. He is married and has two sons and one daughter. Which one of the following is true in relation to screening family members?

- [ ] **A** There is no reason to screen any family member
- [ ] **B** The daughters should not be screened
- [ ] **C** The mother should not be screened
- [ ] **D** The patient's brothers and sisters are probably at a higher risk than his children
- [ ] **E** No screening test is necessary until the children are over 40

116 A 55-year-old secretary has low back pain. X-rays of the spine reveal a generalised decrease in bone density and a compression fracture of the L3 vertebra. The serum calcium concentration is 3 mmol/l. This clinical picture is compatible with which one of the following conditions?

- [ ] **A** Osteoporosis
- [ ] **B** Osteomalacia
- [ ] **C** Multiple myeloma
- [ ] **D** Sarcoidosis
- [ ] **E** Paget's disease

117 A 55-year-old businessman presents with a three month history of epigastric discomfort and weight loss. Physical examination reveals hyperpigmented, non-itchy, heaped-up velvety lesions confined to the axillae and groin. This clinical picture is most compatible with which one of the following conditions?

- [ ] **A** Diabetes mellitus
- [ ] **B** Acromegaly
- [ ] **C** Carcinoma of the stomach
- [ ] **D** Cushing's syndrome
- [ ] **E** Carcinoma of the bronchus

118 A 55-year-old man presents with a six-month history of arthralgia and vasculitic skin rash affecting the lower limbs. Further investigation reveals monoclonal and polyclonal cryoglobulins. This condition is often associated with which one of the following infections?

☐ A   Hepatitis C virus (HCV)
☐ B   Hepatitis B virus (HBV)
☐ C   Epstein–Barr virus (EBV)
☐ D   Parvovirus
☐ E   Cytomegalovirus (CMV)

119 A 45-year-old nurse presents with a three-month history of tinnitus and deafness. A CT scan of the brain shows a well demarcated enhancing mass in the left cerebellopontine angle. Which one of the following is the most likely diagnosis?

☐ A   Medulloblastoma
☐ B   Acoustic neuroma
☐ C   Meningioma
☐ D   Cholesteatoma
☐ E   Haemangioblastoma

120 A 76-year-old man who lives on his own was admitted with general malaise and poor memory. While in hospital a nurse noticed that he is troubled with itching especially at night. Physical examination revealed scratch marks and a thickened linear rash across the wrists and the web spaces between the fingers. Which one of the following is the most appropriate diagnostic measure?

☐ A   The use of a needle to obtain the female mite from the skin lesion
☐ B   Skin biopsy and culture to identify the specific micro-organism
☐ C   Autoantibody screen to exclude a vasculitic disorder
☐ D   Immune staining of a skin biopsy
☐ E   Serum calcium levels to exclude hypercalcaemia

121 A 50-year-old man was admitted with a history of progressive shortness of breath. On checking the blood pressure it was noticed that the systolic blood pressure was detected only during expiration at 120 mmHg. When the cuff pressure was slowly released the systolic blood pressure started to become detectable during both expiration and inspiration at 75 mmHg. Which one of the following clinical conditions is least likely to be associated with this physical sign?

- [ ] **A** Cardiac tamponade
- [ ] **B** Chronic obstructive pulmonary disease
- [ ] **C** Restrictive cardiomyopathy
- [ ] **D** Congestive cardiac failure
- [ ] **E** Constrictive pericarditis

122 A 20-year-old student presents with a three-day history of sore throat, fever and cervical lymphadenopathy. The peripheral blood film shows atypical lymphocytes. Which one of the following tests is most helpful in establishing the diagnosis?

- [ ] **A** Widal's test
- [ ] **B** Paul–Bunnell test
- [ ] **C** Tuberculin test
- [ ] **D** Antinuclear antibodies
- [ ] **E** Rose–Waaler test

123 You see a 35-year-old woman who has been discharged following a successful major neurosurgical procedure for intracranial saccular aneurysm. Further work-up to identify any risk factor for intracranial aneurysm should be focused on each of the following, except

- [ ] **A** Hypertension
- [ ] **B** Autosomal dominant polycystic kidney disease
- [ ] **C** Marfan's syndrome
- [ ] **D** Ehlers–Danlos syndrome
- [ ] **E** Coarctation of the aorta

124 A 55-year-old woman presents with generalised itching of more than six months' duration. Examination of the skin is unremarkable. Which one of the following tests is least helpful in the management of this itching?

- [ ] **A** Antimitochondrial antibodies
- [ ] **B** Serum cholesterol
- [ ] **C** Serum creatinine
- [ ] **D** Haemoglobin
- [ ] **E** Thyroid function test

125 A 91-year-old widow has been in the observation ward of the Emergency Department for 24 hours following a fall. During the night she suddenly becomes confused and agitated, accusing the nurses of being 'Nazis'. She has hit a porter with her walking stick. She scores 3/10 on the Abbreviated Mental Test Score. Physical examination is unremarkable except a pyrexia of 38.5°C and right basal crepitations. Blood gases are normal. A chest X-ray shows right lower lobe shadowing. Which one of the following is the most important initial management?

- [ ] **A** Counselling the patient about her behaviour
- [ ] **B** Intravenous antibiotics
- [ ] **C** Move patient to a well lit single room
- [ ] **D** Loraxepam 50 µg intramuscularly
- [ ] **E** Risperidone 1 mg orally

126 A 25-year-old man who was found to be a carrier for the hereditary haemochromatosis gene asks to see you for further advice. You tell him that there is a chance that he might develop the disease when he is older and that you are going to start regular monitoring to identify early manifestations of the disease. Which one of the following would be the most appropriate first screening test?

- [ ] **A** Hepatic iron concentration
- [ ] **B** Serum ferritin concentration
- [ ] **C** Total iron-binding capacity
- [ ] **D** Serum transferrin saturation
- [ ] **E** Haemoglobin

127 A 63-year-old man presents with excessive bruising on the trunk and both lower limbs. The full blood count is normal but the prothrombin time is prolonged. This man could be suffering with each of the following conditions, except

☑ A Malabsorption with steatorrhoea
☐ B Warfarin overdose
☐ C Factor VII deficiency
☑ D Adrenal failure
☐ E Liver failure

128 A 20-year-old otherwise healthy student presents with fever, headache and photophobia. CSF examination identifies *Neisseria meningitidis*. Each of the following statements are true except

☐ A Treatment with penicillin should be initiated immediately
☐ B It can be prevented by administration of rifampicin
☐ C CSF glucose concentration is usually low
☐ D Deficiencies of late complement components predispose to recurrent episodes of meningococcal meningitis
☐ E Group B vaccine is far more effective than group A or C vaccines

129 A 60-year-old man noticed reduced exercise tolerance and excessive tiredness on minimal exertion. He is known to have diverticular disease of the large bowel. Physical examination shows skin and conjunctival pallor. The haemoglobin was 8 g/dl with a hypochromic and microcytic peripheral blood picture. Which one of the following statements about this condition is true?

☑ A Both serum iron and total iron-binding capacity are reduced
☐ B The bone marrow iron stores are generally maintained
☐ C The reticulocyte count is low in relation to the degree of anaemia
☐ D Serum ferritin levels are increased
☐ E The platelet count is usually reduced

130 A 28-year-old man presents with a two-week history of cough and fever. The chest X-ray shows patchy consolidation in the lower lobe of the right lung. Further tests confirm the diagnosis of *Mycoplasma* pneumonia. Which one of the following antibiotics will be most effective in the treatment of this infection?

- [ ] **A** Vancomycin
- [ ] **B** Metronidazole
- [ ] **C** Tetracycline
- [ ] **D** Ampicillin
- [ ] **E** Aciclovir

131 A 30-year-old woman is referred because of double vision. Neurological examination shows impaired abduction of the right eye, double vision on looking to the right side and an absent light reflex in the right pupil. The most likely diagnosis is

- [ ] **A** Progressive external ophthalmoplegia
- [ ] **B** Posterior communicating artery aneurysm
- [ ] **C** Myasthenia gravis
- [ ] **D** Multiple sclerosis
- [ ] **E** Right third nerve palsy due to diabetes mellitus

132 After isolating a case of meningococcal meningitis in a university campus you are asked to reassure the residents and increase their awareness about the role of airborne spread in disease transmission. Which one of the following examples would you also choose to highlight the importance of airborne spread of disease?

- [ ] **A** Hepatitis A infection
- [ ] **B** Pulmonary tuberculosis
- [ ] **C** AIDS
- [ ] **D** Leprosy
- [ ] **E** Poliomyelitis

133 You advise barrier nursing on the ward for a 60-year-old man with bacillary dysentery. The medical students inquire about the prevention of hospital cross-infection by using barrier nursing. Which one of the following conditions will you choose as a second example to highlight this point?

- [ ] **A** Legionellosis
- [ ] **B** Malaria
- [ ] **C** Typhoid fever
- [ ] **D** Bacterial endocarditis
- [ ] **E** Rheumatic fever

134 A 78-year-old man presents with a two-week history of increasing shortness of breath and ankle swelling. He is known to have congestive cardiac failure (CCF) and is found to have a pleural effusion. The two options for evaluation of his pleural effusion include an empirical trial of diuresis or a diagnostic thoracentesis. Which one of the following clinical findings would suggest that a thoracentesis should be performed first?

- [ ] **A** Fever
- [ ] **B** Symmetrical pleural effusions
- [ ] **C** Cardiomegaly
- [ ] **D** Pleural effusion predominantly on the right side
- [ ] **E** Associated pericardial effusion

135 A 27-year-old lawyer complains of sudden vision loss in the left eye, with no other symptoms. Visual field examination reveals central scotoma in the left eye. Ophthalmoscopy reveals an elevated optic nerve head in the left eye, with no other abnormalities. The most likely diagnosis is

- [ ] **A** Papillitis
- [ ] **B** Central retinal artery occlusion of the left eye
- [ ] **C** Retinal detachment
- [ ] **D** Macular degeneration
- [ ] **E** Papilloedema

136 A 27-year-old man noticed some difficulty in putting on his shirt. He had undergone cervical lymph node biopsy a week earlier. He was unable to shrug his right shoulder. A lesion of which one of the following nerves is the most likely cause of this presentation?

- [ ] **A** Phrenic
- [ ] **B** Glossopharyngeal
- [ ] **C** Spinal accessory
- [ ] **D** Vagus
- [ ] **E** Axillary

137 A 30-year-old woman with gluten-sensitive enteropathy presents with a vesicular rash over the knee and upper back. Which one of the following is the most likely diagnosis?

- [ ] **A** Pemphigoid
- [ ] **B** Dermatitis herpetiformis
- [ ] **C** Bullous pemphigus
- [ ] **D** Psoriasis
- [ ] **E** Lichen planus

138 A 68-year-old man presented with a two-week history of progressive decline in general health, malaise and confusion. Three days prior to his admission to the hospital he became short of breath and was febrile. While in hospital, blood culture grew *Streptococcus bovis* from repeated samples. Each of the following statements are true, except

- [ ] **A** *Streptococcus bovis* is part of the normal oral flora
- [ ] **B** Echoardiogram should be organised immediately
- [ ] **C** Intravenous penicillin G is the treatment of choice
- [ ] **D** *Streptococcus bovis* is a Gram-positive coccus
- [ ] **E** Barium enema would be advised to exclude colonic malignancy

139 A 22-year-old woman presents with weight loss, loose bowel motions and anaemia. Jejunal biopsy shows villous atrophy. Which one of the following statements about this condition is not accurate?

- [ ] **A** This may result from dietary carbohydrate intolerance
- [ ] **B** It is associated with increased serum anti-endomysial antibodies
- [ ] **C** It is associated with vesicular skin rash
- [ ] **D** The bowel lesion is often confined to the proximal small intestine
- [ ] **E** It increases the risk of small bowel lymphoma

140 A 22-year-old woman presented with an erythematous rash on both ear lobes. She was told that this was probably allergic contact dermatitis. This condition is an example of which one of the following types of hypersensitivity reaction?

- [ ] **A** Anaphylactic
- [ ] **B** Cytotoxic
- [ ] **C** Immune complex
- [ ] **D** Cell-mediated delayed response
- [ ] **E** Anaphylactoid

141 The ascitic fluid analysis from a 42-year-old woman who presents with a distended abdomen shows raised protein at 45 g/l. Which one of the following conditions is not likely to be responsible for this woman's illness?

- [ ] **A** Tuberculous peritonitis
- [ ] **B** Meigs' syndrome
- [ ] **C** Budd–Chiari syndrome
- [ ] **D** Peritoneal metastatic disease
- [ ] **E** Constrictive pericarditis

142 A 33-year-old homosexual man presents with cough and rapidly progressive shortness of breath. He is known to have had AIDS for the last two years. Chest X-rays show diffuse, bilateral interstitial infiltrates. Which one of the following is the most appropriate diagnostic approach in this patient?

- [ ] **A** Induced sputum analysis
- [ ] **B** Open lung biopsy
- [ ] **C** Bronchoalveolar lavage
- [ ] **D** Gallium scan
- [ ] **E** Transbronchial lung biopsy

143 A 60-year-old lady with diabetes mellitus is seen in an annual review clinic. You notice multiple oval light-brown atrophic lesions on the shins of both legs, which vary in shape and have an average size of 1 × 2 cm. Which one of the following is the most likely diagnosis?

- [ ] **A** Necrobiosis lipoidica diabeticorum
- [ ] **B** Scleroedema diabeticorum
- [ ] **C** Eruptive xanthoma
- [ ] **D** Diabetic dermopathy
- [ ] **E** Acanthosis nigricans

144 A 33-year-old homosexual man presents with fever, cough and rapidly progressive shortness of breath. He tested positive for HIV. Which one of the following is the most likely cause of this pulmonary infection?

- [ ] **A** Tuberculosis
- [ ] **B** Encapsulated bacteria
- [ ] **C** Histoplasmosis
- [ ] **D** Toxoplasmosis
- [ ] **E** *Pneumocystis carinii*

145 A 73-year-old man presents with sudden onset of right-sided weakness. Physical examination reveals a right carotid bruit and the brain CT scan shows a left internal capsule infarct. Which of the following statements is true?

☐ **A** Ischaemic cerebral infarction is responsible for 80% of strokes

☐ **B** A bruit is a reliable predictor of the degree of stenosis

☐ **C** Atheroma is most commonly seen in the external carotid artery

☐ **D** At his age, the most likely source of cerebral embolism is the heart

☐ **E** Surgery is the only option for patients with complete occlusion of the internal carotid artery

146 The liver function tests of a 53-year-old sailor show normal bilirubin, and slightly raised ALP and ALT. The serum α-fetoprotein is three times above the normal limit. Which one of the following conditions is not associated with raised serum α-fetoprotein?

☐ **A** Hepatocellular carcinoma

☐ **B** Neuroblastoma

☐ **C** Teratoma

☐ **D** Acute hepatitis

☐ **E** Bladder carcinoma

147 A 30-year-old otherwise healthy teacher presents with a two-week history of increasing shortness of breath, orthopnoea and paroxysmal nocturnal dyspnoea. He recalls a week or two of 'flu like illness preceding this episode. The chest X-rays show pulmonary congestion and cardiomegaly. The echocardiogram shows dilated cardiac chambers and an ejection fraction of 20%. The virus most likely responsible for this patient's illness is?

☐ **A** Epstein–Barr virus

☐ **B** Cytomegalovirus

☐ **C** Influenza A virus

☐ **D** Coxsackievirus B

☐ **E** Human immunodeficiency virus (HIV)

148 The number of GP consultations in the first 5 years of life was obtained for a group of 100 children. Their parents were asked to complete a parenting skills questionnaire from which a skills score (an integer value ranging from 0 to 25) was determined. Which one of the following would be the most appropriate method of analysis to assess whether low parenting skills are related to a higher number of GP consultations?

- ☐ **A** Spearman correlation
- ☐ **B** Chi-square test
- ☐ **C** Mann–Whitney U-test
- ☐ **D** Paired *t*-test
- ☐ **E** McNemar's test

149 A 58-year-old woman was in hospital with pneumonia. She was receiving treatment with antibiotics and oxygen. A week later she developed profuse watery diarrhoea and was diagnosed with *Clostridium difficile* infection. She had a similar diagnosis made a year earlier while in hospital with a chest infection. Each of the following statements are true, except

- ☐ **A** Diagnosis of *C. difficile* is most commonly made by cytotoxicity assay
- ☐ **B** Exposure to antibiotics for treatment of other infections is regarded as a risk factor for recurrent *C. difficile* colitis
- ☐ **C** *C. difficile* is part of the normal intestinal flora
- ☐ **D** Punctate plaques on hyperaemic mucosa and patchy yellow membranes are characteristic findings on sigmoidoscopy
- ☐ **E** Approximately 1–2% per year progress to carcinoma

150 A 23-year-old woman presented with a one-week history of cough. In the first two days she coughed up 5 ml of blood on three occasions. The initial laboratory evaluation should include all of the following, except

- ☐ **A** Chest X-rays
- ☐ **B** Full blood cell count (FBC)
- ☐ **C** Sputum for cytology
- ☐ **D** Coagulation studies
- ☐ **E** Spirometry

151 A 68-year-old man presents with progressive weight loss and bone pain. The pain is localised to the shoulders, spine and left upper arm. He describes it as a dull ache, worse at night. X-rays of these areas confirm widespread bone lesions, consistent with bone metastases. The neoplasm least likely to be responsible for this clinical picture is

☐ A Multiple myeloma
☐ B Colorectal cancer
☐ C Lung cancer
☐ D Prostate cancer
☐ E Thyroid cancer

152 A 23-year-old woman who was diagnosed with depression was commenced on Seroxat®. The patient's partner was so dissatisfied with the change in their sex life and the decline in his girlfriend's libido that he asked for the medication to be discontinued. Which one of the following antidepressants has the least adverse effect on sexual functioning?

☐ A Venlafaxine hydrochloride
☐ B Amitriptyline
☐ C Paroxetine hydrochloride
☐ D Bupropion hydrochloride
☐ E Fluoxetine hydrochloride

153 A 63-year-old man with type 2 diabetes who is known to suffer with angina was admitted with severe retrosternal chest pain and vomiting. The 12-lead ECG confirmed an anterior wall Q-wave myocardial infarction. Q-wave myocardial infarction is usually caused by

☐ A Prolonged cardiac muscle spasm
☐ B Cystic medial necrosis
☐ C Thrombus superimposed on pre-existing atherosclerotic plaque
☐ D Coronary vasospasm
☐ E Embolism from aortic debris

154 A 53-year-old obese type 2 diabetic woman who failed a trial of diet to control her diabetes has been treated with metformin for the last three years. However, the Hb A_{1c} on the last three tests was more than 9%. What is the most appropriate next step to maintain adequate glucose control?

☐ A Immediately begin basal-prandial insulin therapy (four injections daily)
☐ B Discontinue the metformin and start another agent of the same or a different class
☐ C Continue with metformin for at least another year to achieve full efficacy
☐ D Continue with metformin and add glipizide
☐ E Continue with metformin and add a thiazolidinedione

155 A 58-year-old woman who has had Sjögren's syndrome for ten years presents with enlarged cervical lymph nodes. Which one of the following is the most likely neoplasm responsible for this presentation?

☐ A Gastric carcinoma
☐ B Lymphoma
☐ C Bronchial carcinoma
☐ D Chronic lymphatic leukaemia
☐ E Pancreatic adenocarcinoma

156 A 54-year-old man has been transferred from the Intensive Care Unit to a rehabilitation ward. He sustained an extensive acute anterior myocardial infarction four months ago. He sustained cardiac arrest and had prolonged cardiopulmonary resuscitation. He was comatose for ten days and then went into a persistent vegetative state (PVS) according to the ICU report. In this clinical state you would expect all the following characteristic features, except

☐ A Preserved sleep–wake cycle
☐ B Inability to speak
☐ C Communication may be possible with blinking eye movements
☐ D Inability to move arms or legs
☐ E No cognitive function

157 A 60-year-old woman is known to have chronic renal failure secondary to chronic glomerulonephritis. She was noted to have raised blood pressure on two visits during the last three months. Physical examination reveals no other cardiovascular abnormalities, the lungs are clear and there is no peripheral oedema. Which one of the following is hypertension in this patient primarily caused by?

- [ ] **A** Elevated renal levels
- [ ] **B** Volume overload
- [ ] **C** Enhanced activity of the sympathetic nervous system
- [ ] **D** Erythropoietin therapy for anaemia
- [ ] **E** Hypercalcaemia from secondary hyperparathyroidism

158 A 20-year-old university student saw her doctor for multiple areas of inflamed acne rash on her face and upper chest. She was given minocycline and advised to use antiseptic lotions and creams. Seven months later her acne has improved but in the last two months she noticed a persistent erythematous rash covering the cheeks and the nose, worse on a sunny day. She also complained of pain in the knees, elbows and wrists with prominent stiffness, myalgia and lethargy. Which one of the following is the most likely diagnosis?

- [ ] **A** Drug-induced systemic lupus erythematosus (SLE)
- [ ] **B** Rheumatoid arthritis
- [ ] **C** Skin lotion-induced urticaria
- [ ] **D** Rheumatic fever
- [ ] **E** Rosacea

159 A 66-year-old woman who frequently notes a sensation of 'food being held up' somewhere behind the 'breastbone' and chest pain is referred for further assessment. She was diagnosed with scleroderma a year ago. Which one of the following would be the most appropriate test at this stage?

- [ ] **A** Chest X-ray
- [ ] **B** Barium swallow
- [ ] **C** CT scan of the chest
- [ ] **D** Oesophagogastroscopy
- [ ] **E** ECG

160 A 56-year-old grossly obese man attends the Outpatient Clinic with his wife. She has noticed that her husband, while sleeping, had ceased to breathe on several occasions and she fears that breathing may not resume on one of these occasions. She also reports loud snoring and gasping. You suspect that he might be suffering from obstructive sleep apnoea syndrome (OSAS). Which one of the following statements about this condition is accurate?

☐ A A definitive diagnosis can be made on the basis of his wife's description and physical examination alone
☐ B All patients with OSAS are obese
☐ C Absence of daytime symptoms is characteristic
☐ D The most effective treatment is continuous positive airway pressure
☐ E Death from acute renal failure is responsible for the high mortality in this disorder

161 A 20-year-old taxi driver presents with persistent cough with copious greenish sputum. Last year he had two episodes of pneumonia and one attack of right otitis media. His past medical history shows that he had similar episodes as a child, at a rate of one or two episodes of upper respiratory tract infection per year. The immunoglobulin levels were low. The total T-cell count and counts of subclasses of T cells are normal. Which one of the following statements is true?

☐ A The most likely underlying disease is chronic granulomatous disease
☐ B The purified protein derivative skin test is expected to be negative
☐ C He should be advised to avoid all live viral vaccines
☐ D For selective IgA deficiency the treatment of choice is intravenous immunoglobulin
☐ E Immunoglobulin replacement is the definitive treatment for common variable immunodeficiency

162 A 50-year-old woman was transferred from a surgical ward to the Intensive Care Unit. She was admitted with abdominal pain, confusion, fever and vomiting. Her temperature was 39°C, pulse 110 bpm and blood pressure 80/40 mmHg. Large bruises covered her skin and after venesection for obtaining a blood sample it was difficult to stop the blood oozing from the puncture site. Blood culture was positive for Gram-negative organisms. Which of the following blood abnormalities is not characteristic of this disorder?

- [ ] **A** Elevated d-dimer levels in the blood
- [ ] **B** Elevated fibrinogen levels
- [ ] **C** Low platelet count
- [ ] **D** Schistocytes on a peripheral blood smear
- [ ] **E** Prolonged activated partial thromboplastin time

163 A 31-year-old otherwise healthy woman has been experiencing slight pain in the right eye, with irritation for six months. On examination she was found to have bilateral proptosis. Which one of the following is the most likely diagnosis?

- [ ] **A** Orbital pseudotumour
- [ ] **B** Graves' disease
- [ ] **C** Optic nerve glioma
- [ ] **D** Cavernous hemangioma
- [ ] **E** Histiocytosis X

164 A 66-year-old heavy smoker notices a gradual decline in his ability to walk the dog. He used to walk four miles every day. Which of the following tests would most reliably establish the diagnosis of chronic obstructive pulmonary disease (COPD)?

- [ ] **A** Peak expiratory flow rate
- [ ] **B** Chest X-ray
- [ ] **C** High-resolution CT scan of the chest
- [ ] **D** ECG
- [ ] **E** Spirometry

165 A 28-year-old soldier based in Saudi Arabia was flown home with a two-week history of fever, headache, general malaise and sweating. He also complains of severe dull backache. Blood cultures were negative. An agglutination test was positive for brucellosis. Each of the following statements is true, except

- [ ] **A** An enlarged spleen may be identified on physical examination
- [ ] **B** Septic discitis causing backache should be considered in this case
- [ ] **C** Contaminated dairy products are the usual source of infection
- [ ] **D** Routine blood cultures are often negative
- [ ] **E** Treatment with penicillin should be initiated without delay

166 A 30-year-old schizophrenic man presented with recurrent spasms in the neck, thought to be a side effect of his antipsychotic medication. Which of the following side effects of antipsychotic drugs are known to be extrapyramidal symptoms?

- [ ] **A** Clasp-knife rigidity
- [ ] **B** Action tremor
- [ ] **C** Festinant gait
- [ ] **D** Diplopia
- [ ] **E** Scanning speech

167 A 60-year-old man was admitted with progressive shortness of breath. He has orthopnoea and paroxysmal nocturnal dyspnoea. His pulse was 100 bpm and blood pressure 80/40 mmHg. There were fine crackles at the bases of both lungs. He received oxygen, diuretics, diamorphine and was nursed propped up in bed. There was no significant improvement and a positive inotropic drug was added. The greatest benefit derived from administering a positive inotropic drug to a patient in heart failure results from

- [ ] **A** A reduction in heart rate
- [ ] **B** A reduction in heart size
- [ ] **C** An increase in end-diastolic pressure
- [ ] **D** An increase in wall thickness
- [ ] **E** An increase in cardiac excitability

168 A 64-year-old man with multiple myeloma was referred because of a rapid decline in his health. He received six courses of cytotoxic drugs and steroid in the last three years. Two weeks ago, while on holiday, he developed a problem with micturition and he underwent intravenous pylography (IVP). The blood urea is 32 mmol/l and the serum creatinine 480 μmol/l. Which one of the following mechanisms is the least likely cause of the impaired renal function?

☐ **A** Primary amyloidosis
☐ **B** Cast nephropathy
☐ **C** Hypercalcaemia
☐ **D** Plasma cell invasion of the kidney
☐ **E** Radiocontrast administration during the IVP test

169 A 57-year-old man with diabetes mellitus was transferred from the Neurology Unit for tighter control of his blood glucose. He was diagnosed with mononeuritis of the left common peroneal nerve. Physical examination of the left leg might reveal each of the following signs, except

☐ **A** Loss of extension of the big toe
☐ **B** Foot-drop
☐ **C** Loss of eversion of the foot
☐ **D** Anaesthesia of the lateral aspect of the leg
☐ **E** Loss of the ankle jerk

170 The bone marrow smear examination from a 60-year-old farmer identified more than 20% of the cellular element to be plasma cells. Which of the following cell types is capable of becoming a plasma cell?

☐ **A** Lymphocyte
☐ **B** Megakaryocyte
☐ **C** Mast cell
☐ **D** Eosinophil
☐ **E** Monocyte

171 The culture and sensitivity result of a wound swab from a 65-year-old diabetic man revealed a Gram-positive organism. Which one of the following tests would best differentiate staphylococcal from streptococcal species?

☐ A Coagulase
☐ B Indole
☐ C Catalase
☐ D Oxidase
☐ E Urease

172 The parathyroid hormone levels from an 80-year-old man with bone pain are significantly elevated. Which one of the following changes in plasma ion concentration is the major stimulus for parathyroid hormone secretion?

☐ A An increase in calcium
☐ B A decrease in calcium
☐ C An increase in sodium
☐ D A decrease in potassium
☐ E An increase in chloride

173 After the first dose of penicillin for cellulitis of the leg a 39-year-old man develops severe shortness of breath and wheeze with a widespread urticarial rash affecting the face and the skin of the trunk. This reaction occurs as the result of mediator release from which one of the following types of cells?

☐ A Antigen-presenting cells
☐ B Mast cells
☐ C Neutrophils
☐ D Monocytes
☐ E Lymphocytes

174 A 77-year-old woman resident in a nursing home presents with severe back pain. She has no significant medical history. X-rays of her spine and pelvis show diffusely decreased bone mass and general laboratory measurements reveal a low calcium level. Which of the following is the most likely cause of this patient's hypocalcaemia?

- [ ] **A** Osteoporosis
- [ ] **B** Multiple myeloma
- [ ] **C** Osteomalacia
- [ ] **D** Chronic renal failure
- [ ] **E** Primary hyperthyroidism

175 The renal function blood tests of a 34-year-old woman show: creatinine 180 μmol/l, urea 6 mmol/l. The patient has no past medical history of significance. The serum creatinine concentration is a suboptimal measure of kidney function because it is affected by each of the following, except

- [ ] **A** Muscle trauma
- [ ] **B** Cefoxitin therapy
- [ ] **C** Late-stage muscular dystrophy
- [ ] **D** High serum lipid levels
- [ ] **E** Pregnancy

176 A 26-year-old man comes to your office concerned about getting chickenpox because he cannot recall having it as a child. He inquires about being vaccinated to prevent chickenpox. Which of the following is the most appropriate advice at this time?

- [ ] **A** All adults are immune to chickenpox
- [ ] **B** He should proceed immediately with varicella vaccination
- [ ] **C** Varicella antibody testing should be performed because it is likely that he is already immune
- [ ] **D** Chickenpox in adults is not a serious illness, so he need not worry about it
- [ ] **E** Varicella vaccination is not indicated for adult males

177 A 43-year-old man is brought to the hospital with a hip fracture following a minor fall. Bone density measurements of the patient's spine and hip reveal osteoporosis. Each of the following serum levels should be measured in this patient, except

- ☐ **A** Potassium levels
- ☐ **B** Serum oestrogen
- ☐ **C** Thyroid function test
- ☐ **D** Serum protein electrophoresis
- ☐ **E** Vitamin D and calcium

178 The 12-lead ECG from a 33-year-old man shows peaked T waves and widened QRS complexes. His plasma potassium level is 7.8 mmol/l. Administration of which one of the following agents is the most appropriate initial therapy?

- ☐ **A** Sodium bicarbonate
- ☐ **B** Insulin plus glucose, intravenously
- ☐ **C** Sodium polystyrene sulfonate, orally
- ☐ **D** Calcium gluconate, intravenously
- ☐ **E** Loop diuretics

179 A 22-year-old pregnant bartender is concerned about the wellbeing of her unborn baby. It transpires that she has a problem with alcohol and that she drinks half a bottle of spirit (brandy) every night and has done so for the last three years. She has continued to drink this amount during the pregnancy. She is 16 weeks pregnant. Which of the following effects on the fetus is a feature of excessive alcohol intake during pregnancy?

- ☐ **A** Bulging eyes
- ☐ **B** Low birth weight
- ☐ **C** Macrocephaly
- ☐ **D** Thick upper lip
- ☐ **E** Prominent maxillary area

180 A 60-year-old woman was referred with retention of urine and weakness in both lower limbs. More recently she has noticed a difference in feeling when wiping herself after a bowel movement. The past medical history revealed a three-month history of unremitting low back pain radiating to both lower limbs. She was walking using a frame. An MRI scan of the spine was arranged to confirm the diagnosis of cauda equina lesion. Each of the following physical signs is characteristic of this lesion, except

- [ ] **A** Weak hip extensors
- [ ] **B** Ankle clonus
- [ ] **C** Saddle (perineal) anaesthesia
- [ ] **D** Lax anal sphincter tone
- [ ] **E** Tenderness on palpating the spine

181 A 40-year-old man has developed pain in the right loin. The pain is colicky in nature. Urinalysis shows microscopic haematuria. Ultrasound examination of the kidneys confirms the diagnosis of a renal stone in the right kidney. Further assessment might identify each of the following as a likely cause of the kidney stone, except

- [ ] **A** Hypercalcaemia
- [ ] **B** Hypercalciuria
- [ ] **C** Hyperuricaemia with gout
- [ ] **D** Hypercitraturia
- [ ] **E** Hyperuricosuria

182 An asymptomatic 19-year-old military recruit has a routine examination on entry to the service. A urine sample showed microalbuminuria. Which one of the following mean albumin excretion results would indicate microalbuminuria?

- [ ] **A** 10 mg/day
- [ ] **B** 20 mg/day
- [ ] **C** 200 mg/day
- [ ] **D** 500 mg/day
- [ ] **E** 1000 mg/day

183　A 20-year-old hairdresser presents with a complaint of having seen 'blood in his urine'. He relates that he had recently had an upper respiratory tract infection. Which one of the following findings is most likely to suggest a non-glomerular source of bleeding?

☐　A　Crenated (dysmorphic) red blood cells
☐　B　Red blood cell casts
☐　C　Lipiduria
☐　D　Proteinuria (> 1 g/24 h) with haematuria
☐　E　Eosinophils in the urine

184　A 20-year-old student presents with a pale puffy face. Physical examination reveals generalised oedema. Which one of the following findings is least consistent with nephrotic syndrome?

☐　A　Haematuria
☐　B　Low serum albumin
☐　C　> 3 g proteinuria/24 h
☐　D　Oval fat bodies in the urine
☐　E　High serum cholesterol

185　A 55-year-old man developed sudden pain in the lower back. He is generally active and jogs for two miles with a friend every day. An intravenous urogram was within normal limits. Dipstick urinalysis was positive for protein. Which one of the following is least likely to give a positive result for protein on dipstick urinalysis?

☐　A　Radiocontrast agents
☐　B　Light chain immunoglobulins in the urine
☐　C　Highly alkaline urine (pH > 8)
☐　D　Urinary infection
☐　E　Exercise

186 A 54-year-old man underwent emergency surgery following acute mesentric artery embolism. The terminal ileum was preserved but 50% of the proximal small bowel was resected. He made full recovery but developed chronic diarrhoea and weight loss. All of the following should be monitored in such a case, except

- [ ] **A** Folic acid
- [ ] **B** Vitamin B$_{12}$
- [ ] **C** Iron
- [ ] **D** Calcium
- [ ] **E** Magnesium

187 A 66-year-old man presents to the Accident and Emergency Department with a two-day history of right anterior, non-radiating chest pain with cough productive of yellow-green red-tinged sputum and a fever of 38.5°C. He has absent breath sounds and bronchial breathing, both anteriorly and at the posterior base of the right lung. Which one of the following tests would be most informative at this time?

- [ ] **A** Full blood count
- [ ] **B** Liver function tests
- [ ] **C** HIV test
- [ ] **D** Thoracentesis
- [ ] **E** Chest X-ray

188 A 60-year-old patient with chronic atrial fibrillation comes to the clinic for his monthly check of the international normalised ratio (INR). He has been taking warfarin 5 mg daily for the past six months. Recently, he was treated for an infection with an antibiotic. He reported a nosebleed early this morning. His vital signs are normal. His full blood count is normal but his INR is 10. Which one of the following would be the best option for his management?

- [ ] **A** Withhold warfarin and monitor INR more frequently
- [ ] **B** Administer vitamin K$_1$ 10 mg by intramuscular injection
- [ ] **C** Administer fresh frozen plasma
- [ ] **D** Withhold warfarin therapy and administer vitamin K$_1$ 3 mg orally
- [ ] **E** Admit the patient to the hospital for observation

189 A 40-year-old woman presents to your clinic with a complaint of generalised itching which has been present off and on for several months but which has recently become more severe and almost constant over the past month. Her physical examination is normal except for obvious excoriations related to scratching. Possible causes of her itching include all of the following, except

☐ A Coeliac sprue
☐ B Dry skin related to a dry winter climate
☐ C Oral contraceptives
☐ D Primary biliary cirrhosis
☐ E Uraemia

190 A 55-year-old woman travelling from England to Australia arrives after an 11-hour flight with a swollen, tender right leg. She does not complain of shortness of breath or chest pain. The only abnormality on physical examination is a swollen right leg up to the knee. A diagnosis of deep vein thrombophlebitis is made and she is admitted to hospital for therapy. Which one of the following regimes should be instituted?

☐ A Start aspirin immediately
☐ B Start warfarin immediately
☐ C Begin oral warfarin and intravenous heparin together
☐ D Begin low molecular weight heparin subcutaneously; begin warfarin on day three
☐ F Begin thrombolytics

191 You are asked to set up a screening service for osteoporosis. A dual-energy X-ray absorptiometry (DEXA) scanner is made available for that reason. In which one of the following groups is it not considered necessary to perform screening for osteoporosis on all members?

☐ A Patients with osteoporosis-related fractures
☐ B Patients with primary biliary cirrhosis
☐ C Men with hypogonadism
☐ D Patients receiving corticosteroids for 16 weeks or more
☐ E Postmenopausal women

192 A 28-year-old man has been referred following an overdose of 100 aspirin tablets. Blood levels reveal a salicylate level of zero. He also claims to have considerable abdominal pain, but does not appear distressed and physical examination reveals no abnormalities except for a number of abdominal scars. The patient is admitted to hospital for observation. Which one of the following would add weight to a diagnosis of Munchausen's syndrome?

- [ ] A The prospect of financial gain from illness
- [ ] B The presence of alcohol dependence
- [ ] C The presence of secondary gain
- [ ] D The presence of true hypochondriasis
- [ ] E The absence of self-inflicted wounds

193 A 44-year-old woman is diagnosed with hepatitis C virus (HCV) infection (genotype 2). She drinks alcohol in excess. The serum ALT level is three times above the upper normal limit and an HCV RNA level is detectable. Which one of the following factors is associated with a slower progression of HCV infection to chronic liver disease?

- [ ] A Older age at infection
- [ ] B Associated HIV infection
- [ ] C HCV genotype 2
- [ ] D Female gender
- [ ] E Alcohol use

194 A 20-year-old man notices excessive bruising whenever he plays football. He remembers that he had unusually heavy bleeding following a tooth extraction at the age of 15. His platelet count is $350 \times 10^9/l$ but the bleeding time is prolonged. Which one of the following bleeding disorders is the most likely diagnosis?

- [ ] A Factor VII deficiency
- [ ] B Haemophilia A
- [ ] C Bernard–Soulier syndrome
- [ ] D Haemophilia B
- [ ] E Idiopathic thrombocytopenic purpura (ITP)

195 A 55-year-old woman with hypercalcaemia is found to have hyperparathyroidism. She reports no fatigue, constipation or weakness. Results of further biochemical blood tests are normal, including indicators of renal function. Which one of the following tests should be ordered next in the evaluation and management of this patient?

☐ A Computed tomography of the neck
☐ B Isotope bone scan
☐ C Dual-energy X-ray absorptiometry (DEXA) bone density measurement
☐ D Ultrasound scan of the parathyroid gland
☐ E Measurement of vitamin D levels

196 A 34-year-old man with a ten-year history of insulin-dependent diabetes mellitus is referred because of difficulties in controlling the blood glucose levels on the current regimen of depot insulin. A previous trial of increasing the insulin dose was complicated by recurrent and sometimes life-threatening hypoglycaemic attacks. He is a shift worker at a local car factory and therefore is finding it hard to comply with the blood glucose monitoring programme. Insulin pump therapy would be appropriate treatment for this patient for all the following reasons, except

☐ A Suboptimal glycaemic control (Hb A_{1c} > 7%)
☐ B Recurrent major hypoglycaemia
☐ C Inability to sense when blood glucose levels are less than 3 mmol/l (ie hypoglycaemic unawareness)
☐ D Unwillingness to monitor his own blood glucose levels
☐ E Being a shift worker

197 As part of an investigative research project looking at the effect of carotid stimulation on the heart, a 24-year-old healthy volunteer was subjected to one minute of pressure on the right carotid artery. This will cause an increase in which one of the following?

☐ A Heart rate
☐ B PR interval
☐ C Ventricular contractility
☐ D Ejection fraction
☐ E Cardiac output

198 A 19-year-old man is taken to his General Practitioner by his mother, who reports a six-month history of weight loss, apathy and poor self care. He dropped out of university soon after starting his course, and now spends most of his time alone in his room playing music. He has recently accused his mother of trying to poison him. At interview he is suspicious and reluctant to talk to you. Select the most likely reason for this presentation.

☐ A Amphetamine misuse
☐ B Depression
☐ C Normal teenage behaviour
☐ D Personality disorder
☐ E Schizophrenia

199 A 15-year-old African boy developed severe watery diarrhoea. A similar disorder has been reported in his village. Cholera was confirmed. Cholera toxin causes diarrhoea by causing

☐ A Secretion of large amounts of chloride in the small intestine
☐ B Inhibition of sodium absorption in the small intestine
☐ C Inhibition of sodium absorption in the colon
☐ D Stimulation of sodium/hydrogen exchange in the small intestine
☐ E Stimulation of sodium/glucose-coupled absorption from the small intestine

200 After a car accident a 28-year-old sales manager loses his memory. The brain region that is most closely associated with amnesia is

☐ A Amygdala
☐ B Occipital lobe
☐ C Precentral gyrus
☐ D Substantia nigra
☐ E Temporal lobe

PAPER THREE QUESTIONS

201 A 19-year-old flight attendant presented with burning and itching around the vagina. Three days later a group of vesicles appeared in that area. She had similar skin lesion six months ago. Further tests confirmed the presence of herpesvirus within these vesicles. Each of the following viruses is regarded as one of the Herpesvirus family, except

- [ ] **A** Smallpox virus
- [ ] **B** Epstein–Barr virus (EBV)
- [ ] **C** Human cytomegalovirus (CMV)
- [ ] **D** Varicella zoster virus (VZV)
- [ ] **E** Herpes simplex type 1 (HSV-1)

202 A 20-year-old bartender planning to find a summer job in Spain asks for your advice about the risk and the best protective measures against excessive exposure to the sun. Which one of the following statements is true?

- [ ] **A** She should stay out of the sun at dawn and sunset to avoid the most harmful UV radiation
- [ ] **B** The risk of systemic lupus erythematosus is significantly increased
- [ ] **C** Vitamin D supplement should be given whenever commercial sunscreens are prescribed
- [ ] **D** Actinic keratosis is more common in fair-skinned individuals
- [ ] **E** Actinic keratosis if not recognised early, will transform into basal cell carcinoma

203 A 28-year-old businessman who flies regularly between London and California was advised to try melatonin supplement orally to ease jet lag symptoms. After a three-week trial he admits to some improvement. Which of the following statements is true about melatonin?

☐ A It improves jet lag symptoms by its unique mild sedative effect
☐ B It is a natural hormone that is secreted by the anterior pituitary gland
☐ C Increased melanin production with grey skin pigmentation might be associated with prolonged use of melatonin in humans
☐ D Its endogenous levels are dramatically reduced on exposure to intense artificial light
☐ E Prolonged use of melatonin might be associated with progeria (early ageing)

204 A 25-year-old woman who takes contraceptive pills presents with swelling of the right leg. Pending a venogram to exclude a possible deep vein thrombosis she is prescribed subcutaneous low molecular weight heparin (LMWH). Which one of the following is the mechanism of action of LMWH?

☐ A Prevents platelet aggregation
☐ B Blocks decarboxylation of vitamin K
☐ C Activates tissue plasminogen
☐ D Inhibits factor Xa
☐ E Depletes factor VII

205 A 40-year-old woman comes to the Dermatology Clinic with an extensive erythematous rash covering the extensor surface of the upper and lower limbs. She has had psoriasis for five years but the disease has generally been mild. She has recently been on holiday to France. Which one of the following is not commonly considered a factor in psoriasis flares?

☐ A Hay fever
☐ B β-Blocker therapy
☐ C HIV infection
☐ D Emotional stress
☐ E Lithium therapy

206 A 33-year-old man presents with blurred vision and photophobia. His eyes are red and the pupils are small. Slit-lamp examination shows evidence of iritis. Each of the following clinical investigations would be helpful in establishing an underlying systemic disease as responsible for his eye problem, except

☐ **A** Chest X-rays
☐ **B** Blood glucose levels
☐ **C** HLA-B27
☐ **D** Purified protein derivatives skin test
☐ **E** Fluorescent treponemal antibody absorption (FTA-ABS) test

207 A 56-year-old factory worker took early retirement on medical grounds. He was diagnosed with carcinoma of the bronchus, which was surgically removed with no evidence of recurrence three years after the surgery. Each of the following represent environmental or occupational carcinogens, except

☐ **A** Radon gas
☐ **B** Polycyclic aromatic hydrocarbons
☐ **C** Toluene diisocyanate
☐ **D** Chloromethyl ether
☐ **E** Asbestos

200 A 45-year-old missionary presented with fever, rigors and excessive sweating. He arrived in the UK three days ago after a three-month humanitarian mission to Africa. Thin and thick blood films were obtained. Each of the following microscopic findings is characteristic of *Plasmodium falciparum* infection, except

☐ **A** Rings appear fine and delicate
☐ **B** Red cells are not enlarged
☐ **C** Crescent-shaped gametocytes
☐ **D** Band forms
☐ **E** Several rings in one RBC

209 A 25-year-old nurse presents with a three-day history of acute-onset polyarthritis, myalgia, fatigue and fever. Physical examination reveals a temperature of 37.8°C, swelling and tenderness at the metacarpophalangeal joints of both hands, and palpable occipital lymph nodes. She had been off work a week earlier nursing her two-year-old son who has a mild febrile illness associated with a red skin rash that covered his cheeks and body. Which one of the following is the most likely cause of her illness?

☐ A Parvovirus B19 infection
☐ B Systemic lupus erythematosus
☐ C Acute rheumatoid arthritis
☐ D Sarcoidosis
☐ E Lyme disease

210 You are asked to see a 35-year-old man who presents to the Emergency Department with palpitations and dizziness. The ECG shows narrow-complex tachycardia at a rate of 160 bpm. You advise adenosine, to be given intravenously, and this results in an immediate termination of the arrhythmia. The mechanism of action of adenosine in the termination of this arrhythmia is through which one of the following?

☐ A Blocking conduction through the atrioventricular (AV) node
☐ B Blocking anterograde conduction over the accessory pathways
☐ C Slowing the rate of sinoatrial (SA) node firing
☐ D Increasing the ventricular threshold for electrical excitability
☐ E Primes the heart for electrical cardioversion

211 You are asked to see a 75-year-old man who presented to the Emergency Department with persistent chest pain. He described the pain as severe and crushing in nature. The pulse was absent in the right radial artery and the blood pressure was 30 mmHg lower in the right arm than in the left one. Dissection of the aorta was suspected. Each of the following features would prompt an immediate surgical referral and possible intervention, except

☐ A Persistent chest pain
☐ B Absent radial pulses
☐ C Involvement of the descending aorta
☐ D CT scan confirming the dissection at the aortic root
☐ E New murmur of aortic regurgitation

212 A 32-year-old woman who presents with headache, photophobia and vomiting has a CT scan of the brain. In considering lumbar puncture, which of the following statements is true?

☐ A It is safe in benign intracranial hypertension
☐ B It is safe if a posterior fossa mass is present
☐ C It is safe if a frontal lobe mass is present
☐ D It is always contraindicated if papilloedema is present
☐ E It is often negative in subarachnoid haemorrhage

213 A 24-year-old man presents complaining of thought block and poor concentration. The most important information from his history that is associated with a significantly increased risk of schizophrenia is

☐ A Being delivered by caesarean section
☐ B A nephew has been diagnosed with schizophrenia
☐ C Being male
☐ D Prior history of substance abuse
☐ E History of childhood attention deficit disorder

214 An outbreak of antibiotic-resistant pneumococcal chest infection is reported in your district. Primary mechanisms of bacterial resistance to antibiotics include each of the following, except

☐ A Gene mutation
☐ B Plasmid transfer
☐ C Intrinsic resistance
☐ D Bacterial biotransformation into virus
☐ E Transposons transfer

215 A 36-year-old man presents with elevated blood pressure (188/112 mmHg, seated) at a yearly physical examination. Previous examinations noted blood pressures of 160/94 mmHg and 158/92 mmHg. On questioning, he admitted episodes, about twice a month, of apprehension, severe headache, perspiration, rapid heartbeat and facial pallor. These episodes had an abrupt onset and lasted 10–15 minutes. Urinary catecholamines adrenaline (epinephrine) and noradrenaline (norepinephrine) are significantly elevated. Which one of the following statements is most accurate about this patient?

☐ A The tumour is definitely localised to the adrenals
☐ B 24-hour ambulatory blood pressure monitoring would confirm white coat syndrome
☐ C Minor tranquillisers in small doses would help to control theses episodes
☐ D Extra-adrenal tumours (paragangliomas) indicate secondary metastasis
☐ E Isotope renogram is essential in establishing the diagnosis

216 A 62-year-old woman is referred for evaluation of progressive exertional dyspnoea and fatigue over the past two years. Examination revealed a grade 3/6 systolic murmur along the left sternal border and bilateral fine crepitations at the lung bases. The natriuretic peptides levels were 20 times the upper limit of normal values. The physiological effects of cardiac natriuretic peptides include each of the following, except

- [ ] A Increase in the glomerular filtration rate
- [ ] B Increased cardiac preload
- [ ] C Decreased aldosterone secretion
- [ ] D Renin–angiotensin system inhibition
- [ ] E Lowering of the blood pressure

217 A 36-year-old woman known to have arthritis of the small joints of the hands for three years is referred for further assessment. Physical examination reveals swan-neck deformity and ulnar deviation. The rheumatoid factor is positive at 1/256 and the ANA is positive at 1/1000 (homogeneous pattern). Which one of the following radiological findings on plain X-rays of the hands would help to differentiate between rheumatoid arthritis and systemic lupus erythematosus (SLE)?

- [ ] A Loss of joint space
- [ ] B Juxtarticular osteoporosis
- [ ] C Subluxaton at the metacarpophalangeal (MCP) joints
- [ ] D Erosions
- [ ] E Soft tissue swelling at the proximal interphalangeal (PIP) joints of the hands

218 A 70-year-old man presents with sudden onset of confusion and vomiting. He is found to have a lower urinary tract infection and is given antibiotics. Which one of the following best explains a decrease in the effective levels of antimicrobials in the elderly?

- [ ] A Altered gastric motility
- [ ] B Decreased absorptive surface
- [ ] C Increase in adipose tissue
- [ ] D Decreased protein binding
- [ ] E Decreased biliary excretion

219 A 66-year-old man had noticed irritation and watering of his left
     eye and saliva dripping from the angle of his mouth. Late in the
     afternoon he developed a progressive ipsilateral facial weakness
     and hyperacusis. Facial nerve palsy is associated with which one
     of the following infectious etiologies?

     ☐ A   HIV infection
     ☑ B   Mumps virus
     ☐ C   *Borrelia burgdorferi*
     ☐ D   *Staphylococcus aureus*
     ☐ E   Cytomegalovirus (CMV)

220 A 30-year-old man is referred for a further opinion. He complains
     of shortness of breath, cough and low-grade fever. Which one of
     the following radiological findings is most suggestive of
     sarcoidosis?

     ☐ A   Massive left-sided pleural effusion
     ☐ B   Lung parenchymal disease and no evidence of
            lymphadenopathy
     ☐ C   Recent chest X-ray shows hilar lymphadenopathy but
            previous reports show only longstanding pulmonary fibrosis
     ☐ D   Isolated mediastinal lymphadenopathy
     ☐ E   Unilateral hilar lymphadenopathy

221 A 27-year-old woman presents with a three-day history of
     pleuritic chest pain. She has been taking contraceptive pills.
     Physical examination of the lower limbs is normal. The 12-lead
     ECG shows sinus tachycardia and the V/Q scan shows multiple
     mismatched segmental defects in both lung fields. Which one of
     the following statements is not accurate?

     ☐ A   In patients with pulmonary embolism, only 10–20% have
            clinical evidence of deep venous thrombosis
     ☐ B   The S1, Q3, T3 changes on the 12-lead ECG, when
            identified, are diagnostic
     ☐ C   Arterial blood gases are normal in 50% of patients
     ☐ D   Warfarin should be continued for six months
     ☐ E   Thrombolysis should be considered if evidence of
            haemodynamic instability is present

222 A 19-year-old woman is admitted in an emaciated state. Her body mass index is 16 and she has amenorrhoea. A diagnosis of anorexia nervosa has been made. Which of the following abnormalities might you expect on investigation?

- [ ] **A** Low cortisol levels
- [ ] **B** Increased gonadotrophin levels
- [ ] **C** Increased growth hormone levels
- [ ] **D** Increased thyroid stimulating hormone (TSH) levels
- [ ] **E** Increased triiodothyronine (T3) levels

223 You are asked to review a 65-year-old man who was referred because of persistent cough, progressive shortness of breath and weight loss. The chest X-rays show a right apical cavity with a small pleural effusion. The cANCA is strongly positive. At this stage the best course of action is to

- [ ] **A** Initiate steroid therapy 60 mg orally and oral cyclophosphamide
- [ ] **B** Order a proteinase 3 (PR3) antibodies ELISA test
- [ ] **C** Start intravenous cyclphosphamide infusion and oral steroid
- [ ] **D** Perform a tuberculin test
- [ ] **E** Ask for CT scan of the chest

224 You are asked to review a 35-year-old woman who was referred because of persistent cough, progressive shortness of breath and weight loss. The urine sedimentation reveals microscopic haematuria. The chest X-rays show a right apical cavity with small pleural effusion. Each of the following disorders could be the disease behind this presentation, except

- [ ] **A** Sarcoidosis
- [ ] **B** Wegener's granulomatosis
- [ ] **C** Tuberculosis
- [ ] **D** Lymphoma
- [ ] **E** Goodpasture's syndrome

225 A 66-year-old man is referred because his INR is 7.0. He is on warfarin for persistent atrial fibrillation. There is no history of bleeding. Physical examination reveals two small bruises on the anterior part of the right leg. After stopping the warfarin the most appropriate course of action is to

- [ ] A Give phytomenadione 0.5 mg orally for three days
- [ ] B Give fresh frozen plasma 15 ml/kg
- [ ] C Give protamine sulphate intravenously
- [ ] D Give one unit of prothrombin concentrate
- [ ] E Give no treatment but restart warfarin when INR < 5.0

226 A 22-year-old man is found in the street by the police and brought to the Emergency Department. He is semi-naked and has been approaching passers-by in an agitated fashion. Which one of the following statements by the patient most strongly suggests the presence of schizophrenia?

- [ ] A 'All the police in this town have been spying on me'
- [ ] B 'They control me; they made me take my clothes off'
- [ ] C 'I have been given special powers by god to eliminate the anti-Christ'
- [ ] D 'If you don't let me go I'll kill myself'
- [ ] E 'The salaam transputer has degenerated my brain'

227 A 63-year-old man presents with fever and dysuria. Urine culture grew micro-organisms sensitive to quinolones. This group of antibiotics exerts their antimicrobial activities through

- [ ] A Inhibiting gyrase enzymes
- [ ] B Inhibiting β-lactamase enzymes
- [ ] C Inhibiting dihydrofolate reductase enzymes
- [ ] D Inhibiting bacterial ribosomes
- [ ] E Inhibiting cell wall synthesis

228 A 63-year-old man presents with severe chest pain of two hours'
duration. Acute myocardial infarction is confirmed. After the first
24 hours each of the following changes on blood tests might be
encountered, except

☐ **A** Elevated C-reactive protein (CRP)
☐ **B** Raised white cell count
☐ **C** Higher cholesterol levels
☐ **D** Raised d-dimers
☑ **E** Raised myoglobin

229 A husband has noticed a progressive intellectual decline in his
67-year-old wife during the last six months. He says she forgets
their address, telephone number and, on many occasions, their
children's names. He also says that she sees flowers and other
objects on tables or walls when they are not there. Physical
examination reveals a shuffling gait and hand tremor. The Mini
Mental State Examination score is significantly reduced. The
most likely diagnosis is

☐ **A** Alzheimer's disease
☐ **B** Picks disease
☐ **C** Schizophrenia
☑ **D** Lewy body dementia
☐ **E** Depression

230 A 77-year-old man presents with progressive weakness and
wasting of the small muscles of the hands. On examination
widespread fasciculation is noted in the deltoid and vastus
medialis muscles. Brisk reflexes and ankle clonus are present.
The following neuromuscular functions often remain intact in
this condition, except

☑ **A** Intellect
☑ **B** Speech
☐ **C** Sphincter function
☐ **D** Extra-ocular muscle movement
☐ **E** Pinprick sensation

231 A 71-year-old man presents with progressive weakness and wasting of the small muscles of the hands. On examination, there are brisk reflexes in the upper and lower limbs, and widespread fasciculations are also noted in the deltoid and vastus medialis muscles. The most appropriate investigation at this stage is

- [ ] **A** Electromyography and nerve conduction studies
- [ ] **B** Creatine kinase (CK) muscle enzymes
- [ ] **C** Magnetic resonance scan of the brain
- [ ] **D** Cerebrospinal fluid protein analysis
- [ ] **E** Visual-evoked potential

232 A 60-year-old man with no significant medical history presented to the Emergency Department, reporting a first episode of light-headedness on standing up that morning. An ECG showed atrial fibrillation with a heart rate of 150 bpm. He was treated aggressively with intravenous digoxin and, while he was still in the department, he converted to normal sinus rhythm and his heart rate slowed to 62 bpm. The most appropriate course of action at this stage is

- [ ] **A** Continue with oral digoxin
- [ ] **B** Start warfarin therapy
- [ ] **C** Start sotalol 40 mg
- [ ] **D** Stop iv digoxin and monitor
- [ ] **E** Start aspirin 75 mg daily

233 A 40-year-old woman is referred for evaluation of progressive exertional dyspnoea and fatigue over the past two years. Examination reveals a grade 3/6 systolic murmur along the left sternal border and at the apex. An ECG shows atrial fibrillation with a heart rate of 110 bpm. The diagnosis of obstructive hypertrophic cardiomyopathy (HCM) is established by two-dimensional and Doppler echocardiography. Each of the following drugs is regarded as appropriate treatment for this condition, except

- [ ] **A** Digoxin
- [ ] **B** Amiodarone
- [ ] **C** Atenolol
- [ ] **D** Verapamil
- [ ] **E** Disopyramide

234 A 79-year-old man was brought to the Emergency Department after having been found by the police wandering on the street. The patient's medical history was unremarkable except for hyperlipidaemia. After thorough assessment he was found to have poor cognitive function and a reduced Mini Mental State Examination score. The rest of the physical examination was within normal limits, apart from an equivocal right plantar reflex. At this stage each of the following tests would be considered appropriate, except

- [ ] **A** Thyroid function tests
- [ ] **B** Vitamin B_{12} levels
- [ ] **C** Iron and serum ferritin
- [ ] **D** Brain CT scan
- [ ] **E** Enzyme immunoassay (EIA) test for antitreponemal IgG

235 A 78-year-old woman presents with a two-week history of increasing pain in the back. She denies any history of trauma or fall. Physical examination reveals dorsal kyphosis and localised tenderness at T8–T9 vertebrae. The plain radiographs of the spine show a wedge fracture at the T8–T9 vertebrae and generalised reduction in spine bone density. She is started on alendronate 70 mg weekly. Alendronate's mechanism of action is best described as

- [ ] **A** Anabolic
- [ ] **B** Anti-resorptive
- [ ] **C** Oestrogen receptor agonist
- [ ] **D** Selective oestrogen receptor modulator
- [ ] **E** Oestrogen receptor antagonist

236 A 33-year-old man presents with fixed flexion deformities and recurrent painful spasms in both legs. He had a car accident ten years ago that left him paraplegic. Neurological examination reveals upper motor neurone signs with severe spasticity and clonus in both legs. Baclofen helped to ease his spasms and improve the spasticity. Baclofen exerts its action through which one of the following mechanisms?

☐ A α_2-Adrenergic agonist activity
☐ B As γ-aminobutyric acid analogue
☐ C Prevention of calcium ion release at the sarcoplasmic reticulum
☐ D Selective serotonin uptake inhibition
☐ E Selective oestrogen receptor modulation

237 A 75-year-old man presents with a three-week history of recurrent early morning headache and vomiting. Computed tomography of the brain shows multiple opacities with surrounding interstitial oedema in both hemispheres. Which of the following is the least likely primary tumour responsible for the secondary brain metastases?

☐ A Carcinoma of the prostate
☐ B Carcinoma of the bronchus
☐ C Carcinoma of the colon
☐ D Melanoma of the skin
☐ E Thyroid carcinoma

238 A 25-year-old drug representative underwent colonoscopy as part of a family screen. Multiple adenomatous polyps (around 100) were noted in the colon. There were no polyps in the small intestine. His father, who had had a total colectomy, had a similar problem. Which one of the following statements about this patient is most true?

☐ A The risk of development of colon cancer is nearly 100% by the age of 40
☐ B The disorder is inherited in an autosomal recessive pattern
☐ C Mucocutanous pigmentation is often helpful in alerting to the diagnosis
☐ D Total colectomy is reserved for symptomatic patients
☐ E Polypectomy is considered the mainstay of treatment

239 A 45-year-old known heavy drinker presented to the Emergency Department with haematemesis and melaena. He was given a blood transfusion and underwent gastroscopy which confirmed the diagnosis of bleeding oesophageal varices. The varices were injected and no further blood loss was reported. Prophylaxis against future variceal bleeding would include each of the following therapies, except

☐ A Long-term proton pump inhibitor
☐ B Long-term propranolol
☐ C Long-term nitrate therapy
☐ D Serial injections of the varices
☐ E Transjugular intrahepatic portosystemic shunt (TIPS)

240 A 75-year-old woman with long-standing osteoarthritis of the knee is referred for improvement in pain control. You replace her long-term non-steroidal anti-inflammatory drug (NSAID) therapy (diclofenac) with rofecoxib, a cyclo-oxygenase-2 (COX-2) inhibitor. Which one of the following is not considered an indication for the use of COX-2 inhibitors?

☐ A Osteoarthritis of the knee
☐ B Age over 65 years
☐ C Poor response to the traditional NSAIDs
☐ D Previous history of upper gastrointestinal symptoms
☐ E Patients on long-term maximum dose of traditional NSAIDs

241 A 25-year-old woman presents with a one-week history of multiple erythematous tender nodules at the front of both legs. She also complains of general malaise, arthralgia and fatigue. The most helpful single test at this stage is

☐ A Chest X-ray
☐ B Skin biopsy
☐ C Antinuclear antibodies (ANA)
☐ D Anti-neutrophil cytoplasmic antibodies (ANCA)
☐ E HIV test

242 A 44-year-old woman is referred to the Department of Gastroenterology for a 'further opinion' having developed constant peri-umbilical pain radiating to both legs. In the past five years she has been seen by colleagues in neurology, cardiology, rheumatology and endocrinology with a variety of symptoms, including fatigue, back pain, chest pain and joint pain and despite intensive investigations no cause has been identified. Which one of the following is the most likely diagnosis?

- [ ] **A** Conversion disorder
- [ ] **B** Hypochondriasis
- [ ] **C** Somatization disorder
- [ ] **D** Undifferentiated somatoform disorder
- [ ] **E** Depression

243 A 62-year-old man had an anterior wall myocardial infarction and coronary bypass surgery two years ago. He had a 50 pack per year smoking history until two years ago. On further questioning, the patient admits to discontinuing his jogging and tennis over the previous couple of months because of decreased stamina and shortness of breath. He is comfortable at rest. The brain natriuretic peptide (BNP) is significantly elevated. All the following is true for BNP, except

- [ ] **A** A normal BNP level can help exclude heart failure
- [ ] **B** High levels are diagnostic of heart failure
- [ ] **C** Secreted in response to increased ventricular volume
- [ ] **D** Secreted in response to increased ventricular pressure
- [ ] **E** A declining BNP indicates a good response to therapy

244 A 26-year-old woman presents with a history of abdominal pain and chronic diarrhoea for six months. She has lost 5 kg in weight. Examination of the abdomen reveals mild tenderness around the umbilicus. Small intestine biopsy shows mononuclear cell infiltration of the lamina propria and complete villous atrophy. The most likely diagnosis is

- [ ] **A** Coeliac disease
- [ ] **B** Ulcerative colitis
- [ ] **C** Crohn's disease
- [ ] **D** Intestinal lymphoma
- [ ] **E** Villous adenoma

245 A 55-year-old housewife is referred because of excessive tiredness and generalised pain. Physical examination reveals multiple 'tender points' around the neck, anterior chest, elbows and hip region. The most likely diagnosis is

- [ ] **A** Becker's muscular dystrophy
- [ ] **B** Myasthenia gravis
- [ ] **C** Fibromyalgia
- [ ] **D** Duchenne muscular dystrophy
- [ ] **E** Polymyalgia rheumatica

246 A 56-year-old woman has recently been diagnosed with carcinoma of the bronchus. The histopathology report confirms the diagnosis of non-small cell carcinoma. The patient is short of breath and having recurrent haemoptysis. Each of the following features will render surgery inappropriate, except

- [ ] **A** Mediastinal lymphadenopathy
- [ ] **B** Malignant pleural effusion
- [ ] **C** Pathological fracture of the rib
- [ ] **D** Tumour size more than 3 cm
- [ ] **E** FEV_1 less than 0.5 litre

247 A 22-year-old army cadet was dispatched to Cyprus. While there he engaged on several occasions in unprotected sexual intercourse with a female bartender. He was told that she is probably HIV-positive. Each of the following features might indicate seroconversion in this man, except

- [ ] **A** Fever
- [ ] **B** Cervical lymphadenopathy
- [ ] **C** Maculopapular skin rash over the extremities
- [ ] **D** Acute diarrhoea
- [ ] **E** Myalgia

248 A 22-year-old woman presents with sudden onset of severe weakness in both upper and lower limbs. She is bedridden. Her husband claims that she was playing tennis the day before. He admits that recently she has complained of palpitations and has suffered progressive weight loss despite having a very good appetite. Physical examination reveals a 3 × 2.5 cm firm nodule in the left lobe of the thyroid and 2/5 weakness in the upper and lower limbs. The reflexes are diminished but the sensation is intact. Which one of the following is the most likely diagnosis?

☐ A Familial periodic paralysis
☐ B Guillain–Barré syndrome
☐ C Myasthenia gravis
☐ D Eaton–Lambert syndrome
☐ E Cerebrovascular accident

249 A 20-year-old social worker was prescribed amoxicillin for gingivitis by her dentist. Three days later she developed fever and a diffuse skin rash covering the distal part of the extremities. The renal function showed raised urea and creatinine. Which one of the following tests is considered the gold standard for the diagnosis of acute interstitial nephritis?

☐ A Urine eosinophil count
☐ B Renal biopsy
☐ C Gallium-67 scanning
☐ D Renal ultrasonography
☐ E Urine red cells casts

250 A 58-year-old man was in good health until he noted a single episode of sweating, light headedness and near-syncope while walking to his car. He sought emergency care. He denies having fever, chills, dyspnoea, cough, haemoptysis or weight loss. The patient's medical history was unremarkable except for hyperlipidaemia. A chest X-ray demonstrated an anterior mediastinal fullness. A chest CT confirmed an anterior mediastinal mass. Which one of the following is the least likely diagnosis?

☐ A Thymoma
☐ B Teratoma
☐ C Lymphoma
☐ D Goitre
☐ E Neuroblastoma

251 A 44-year-old woman volunteered in a study at a research centre. She was found to have a raised plasma B-type or brain natriuretic peptide (BNP) levels. The major source of plasma BNP secretion in humans is

☐ A Brain
☐ B Atrium
☐ C Ventricle (cardiac)
☐ D Adrenals
☐ E Kidneys

252 You are asked to review a 25-year-old, otherwise healthy woman who complains of daily, persistent, widespread muscle aches and occasional cramps, and has a sustained high creatine kinase over 200 U/l (normal range < 120 U/l). Each of the following investigations is essential in identifying a possible underlying cause for this problem, except

☐ A Thyroid function tests
☐ B Electromyography
☐ C 9-am plasma cortisol
☐ D Serum potassium
☐ E Muscle biopsy

253 You are called to the ward as the nursing staff are concerned that a
34-year-old male patient has been standing in the ward office for an
hour and is refusing to move. You find that the patient is alert but
unresponsive. You attempt to examine the patient. Which of the
following motor disturbances would lead you to suspect catatonia?

☐ A Reduced tone
☐ B Catalepsy
☐ C Cataplexy
☐ D Stereotypy
☐ E Mannerisms

254 A 62-year-old man with a long-standing diabetic nephropathy and
nephrotic syndrome presented to the Emergency Department
because of a two-day history of a swollen right leg. Venography
confirmed the presence of deep vein thrombosis in the right femoral
vein. Which one of the following is the least likely contributing factor
to the development of venous thrombosis in this patient?

☐ A Mutation of factor V Leiden
☐ B Depression of fibrinolysis
☐ C Increased urinary loss of antithrombin III
☐ D Elevated von Willebrand factor
☐ E Platelet hyperaggregation

255 A 25-year-old obese woman was evaluated for headaches, blurred
vision, light-headedness and occasional vomiting of seven
months' duration. Neurological examination revealed marked
bilateral papilloedema. A 2/6 systolic murmur was heard at the left
sternal border. Chest X-rays and computed tomography of the
brain revealed no abnormal findings. Lumbar puncture showed an
opening pressure of 45 cmH$_2$O (normal range 5–8 cmH$_2$O).
Cerebrospinal fluid glucose, protein, cell count, fungal serology,
Gram stain, and culture were all negative. At this point, which one
of the following is the most likely cause of the headaches?

☐ A Chronic meningitis
☐ B Sleep apnoea
☐ C Benign intracranial hypertension
☐ D Temporal arteritis
☐ E Complicated migraine

256 A 43-year-old man presents with haematemesis and melaena. He drinks four to six cans of beer over the weekends. Further investigations confirm the diagnosis of portal vein thrombosis and bleeding osephageal varices. A thrombophilia screen shows increased homocysteine levels. Elevated plasma homocysteine is also known to be associated with each of the following situations/disorders, except

☐ A Heavy smoking
☐ B Chronic alcoholism
☐ C Renal failure
☐ D Vitamin B$_{12}$ deficiency
☐ E Hypercholesterolaemia

257 A 25-year-old journalist who had no remarkable medical history presented to a local Emergency Department with symmetrical numbness, tingling and weakness in all four limbs that had been worsening over the past two weeks. The weakness had progressed to the point that the patient could no longer stand up or raise her arms. Laboratory tests done on admission revealed: K$^+$ 1.5 mmol/l, chloride 114 mmol/l, bicarbonate (venous) 15 mmol/l, anion gap 11 mmol/l, Ca^{2+} 2.63 mmol/l and magnesium 1.23 mmol/l. Blood gases showed: Pao$_2$ 12 kPa, Paco$_2$ 4 kPa, pH 7.31. The urinary pH was 7.0. Based on the presentation described, which one of the following is the most likely diagnosis for this patient?

☐ A Cerebrovascular accident
☐ B Thiazide diuretic abuse
☐ C Bulimia nervosa with repeated vomiting
☐ D Guillain–Barré syndrome
☐ E Renal tubular acidosis

258 A couple attend the fertility clinic for further evaluation. They have been married for two years and attempts to conceive have failed so far. They are in their thirties and have no past medical history of note. The wife has one child from a previous marriage. The husband has a previous history of knee surgery for a sport injury and has had anosmia for many years. The most likely cause of infertility is

☐ A Kallmann's syndrome
☐ B Kartagener's syndrome
☐ C Young's syndrome
☐ D Klinefelter's syndrome
☐ E Diabetes mellitus

259 A 39-year-old school secretary was admitted with two episodes of grand mal fits. The patient's medical history was unremarkable except for a fibroid uterus. She had been to India recently on holiday for two weeks but denied having any illness while on holiday. Computed tomography (CT) of the brain showed a 3 × 4 cm tumour at the surface of the right parietal lobe. The tumour had a well-defined margin and was surrounded by interstitial oedema. The overlying inner border of the skull showed evidence of hyperosteosis. The most likely underlying cause for this patient's seizures is

☐ A Arteriovenous malformation
☐ B Tuberculoma
☐ C Cerebral malaria
☐ D Meningioma
☐ E Cysticercosis

260 A 47-year-old alcoholic man is admitted to hospital because he is extremely weak and cannot walk. He has a long history of alcohol abuse, consuming 12 beers per day for over 25 years. He has experienced progressive unsteadiness on his feet with episodes of falling. He cannot fully recall the events before or during his hospital stay. Investigation reveals the following: Na$^+$ 127 mmol/l, urea 100 mmol/l, bilirubin 30 mmol/l, ALT 70 U/l, GGT 140 U/l. Which one of the following is the most likely diagnosis?

  ☐ A Alcoholic vestibular neuronitis
  ☐ B Cerebellar infarction
  ☐ C Subdural haematoma
  ☐ D Central pontine myelinolysis
  ☐ E Wernicke's encephalopathy

261 In the protocol for a proposed clinical trial to assess the effect of including a bran supplement in the diet to reduce symptoms of irritable bowel syndrome (IBS), among patients with a severe form of the disease, the sample size was justified as follows:
"The study would have 90% power to detect a 2-unit difference in global well-being score between the control and intervention group, assuming a standard deviation of 1 unit, and assuming a two-sample t-test is used to compare the scores of the two groups, with a 1% significance level"
In which one of the following circumstances would the proposed sample size need to be increased?

  ☐ A An increase in the stated detectable difference
  ☐ B A decrease in the proposed type II error
  ☐ C A decrease in the incidence of IBS
  ☐ D An increase in the significance level
  ☐ E A decrease in power to 80%

262 A 60-year-old man is admitted with progressive shortness of breath. He has orthopnoea and paroxysmal nocturnal dyspnoea. His pulse is 100 bpm and blood pressure is 180/99 mmHg. A short ejection systolic murmur is heard in the left parasternal area. Which one of the following conditions causes the pulse pressure to increase?

- [ ] **A** Haemorrhage
- [ ] **B** Hypertension
- [ ] **C** Tachycardia
- [x] **D** Heart failure
- [ ] **E** Aortic stenosis

263 A 69-year-old woman was brought by ambulance to the Emergency Department with recurrent tonic–clonic seizures. Her husband said that she had been suffering with early morning headache and vomiting for eight weeks. She was confused and generally weak. Urgent computed tomography of the brain showed multiple contrast-enhanced deposits through both hemispheres, with surrounding interstitial oedema. Dexamethasone was given intravenously, with rapid improvement in muscle power, mobility and level of consciousness. Which one of the following tests has the greatest chance of identifying the site of the primary tumour?

- [ ] **A** Chest X-ray
- [ ] **B** Ultrasound of the kidneys
- [ ] **C** Sigmoidoscopy
- [ ] **D** Ultrasound of the thyroid gland
- [x] **E** Mammography of the breast

264 An 18-year-old woman is admitted early in the morning having taken a paracetamol overdose. She claimed that she ingested 30 tablets following an argument with her boyfriend the night before at around 10 pm. She denied having any abdominal pain, nausea or vomiting. The plasma paracetamol concentration was above the treatment line at eight hours and so an acetylcysteine infusion was given. Each of the following test results 24 hours after the overdose should prompt you to contact the specialist liver unit, except

☐ A INR > 2
☐ B Serum albumin < 25 g/l
☐ C Blood pH < 7.3
☐ D Serum creatinine concentration > 300 μmol/l
☐ E ALT > 1000 U/l

265 A 69-year-old man has been referred to receive chemotherapy for small cell carcinoma of the bronchus. He was prescribed ondansetron to combat expected nausea and vomiting. Each of the following anti-emetics listed acts centrally at the chemoreceptor trigger zone in the brain, except

☐ A Metoclopramide
☐ B Ondansetron
☐ C Scopolamine
☐ D Haloperidol
☐ E Prochlorperazine

266 A 77-year-old man presented with diffuse pain all over the body, worse at night and on movement. He was not able to sleep for the previous two nights. He is known to have carcinoma of the prostate with bone metastases. In an attempt to control his pain he was given paracetamol and non-steroidal anti-inflammatory drugs initially. Dihydrocodeine was added a week later. Despite initial improvement he continues to have severe bone pain. You consider adding a strong opioid. Which one of the following statements is not true about initiating this treatment?

☐ A Oral administration is the route of choice
☐ B The total daily dose of morphine should not exceed 500 mg
☐ C Sedation associated with morphine use usually abates after five to seven days
☐ D Morphine is seldom helpful in the management of painful muscle spasm
☐ E Haloperidol 1.5 mg at night is useful in controlling opioid-induced nausea or vomiting

267 A 69-year-old man is referred because of a three-day history of passing black stools. He denied any other symptoms. He also denied any history of upper gastrointestinal problem or any history of drinking alcohol. He has taken warfarin 3 mg daily for the last three years for atrial fibrillation and two minor strokes. The international normalised ratio (INR) was within the therapeutic range at 2.2 (target therapeutic range 2–3). The pulse was 80 bpm and regular, blood pressure 130/80 mmHg. His haemoglobin remained above 11 g/dl. The warfarin was stopped and two days later his melaena resolved completely. The most appropriate course of action at this stage is to

☐ A Prescribe long-term clopidogrel 75 mg tablets and avoid using warfarin in the future
☐ B Resume warfarin therapy with a proton pump inhibitor and aim at INR levels between 1.5 and 2.5
☐ C Arrange gastroscopy before starting anticoagulation
☐ D Arrange an echocardiogram to assess the need for further anticoagulation
☐ E Start subcutaneous low molecular weight heparin for ten days and if there is no evidence of recurrence of melaena, reintroduce warfarin but at a smaller dose

268 A 42-year-old woman was referred for evaluation of progressive exertional dyspnoea and fatigue over the past year. The past medical history was unremarkable apart from a recent business trip to India. Examination revealed conjunctival pallor and splenomegaly of 14 cm. Investigations showed: haemoglobin 10.2 g/dl, WBC count 300 $\times$ 10^9/l, with a differential count of neutrophils 44%, metamyelocytes 26%, promyelocytes 18%, basophils 6% and eosinophils 6% and a platelet count of 638 $\times$ 10^9/l. Which one of the following is the most likely diagnosis?

- [ ] **A** Multiple myeloma
- [ ] **B** Lymphoma
- [ ] **C** Malaria
- [ ] **D** Chronic myeloid leukaemia
- [ ] **E** Essential thrombocytopenia

269 A 23-year-old woman was referred for evaluation of anaemia. She has been suffering from irregular menstrual bleeding with heavy periods. Her haemoglobin was 10.6 g/dl with a hypochromic and microcytic peripheral blood picture. She was prescribed iron tablets and given dietary advice about iron-rich food. Which one of the following statements about iron metabolism is not true?

- [ ] **A** Iron is mainly absorbed in the duodenum and upper jejunum
- [ ] **B** Only 10% of the normal dietary iron is absorbed each day
- [ ] **C** Citrate and ascorbate can form complexes with iron that increase absorption
- [ ] **D** Increased absorption is stimulated by hypoxia
- [ ] **E** Iron is initially stored as transferrin

270   You are asked to review a 45-year-old woman who presents with a two-year history of involuntary movements. The movement interferes with her daily activities. She retired from her job as an executive secretary at the age of 43. She was reportedly making some errors at work. She has nothing of note in her past medical or family history. She has been taking phenothiazine for the last six months. Initial neurological examination is notable for generalised choreic movements involving facial as well as limb muscles. Prominent head nodding and tongue protrusion is also noted. Tendon reflexes were 2+ and equal with down-going plantars. There was some difficulty with serial subtractions, and thinking was illogical and tangential at times. Which one of the following is the most likely diagnosis?

- ☑ **A** Huntington's disease
- ☐ **B** Parkinson's disease
- ☐ **C** Dystonic reaction to phenothiazines
- ☐ **D** Tardive dyskinesia
- ☐ **E** Sydenham's chorea

271   You are asked to see a 45-year-old car salesman who presented with sudden onset of fever, headache, confusion and behavioural changes. His family reported that he had two epileptic fits on the way to hospital. He drinks four cans of beer at the weekend. He travels twice a year to India to promote his business. Magnetic resonance imaging of the brain shows changes in the medial temporal areas bilaterally. Cerebrospinal fluid (CSF) analysis reveals abundant RBCs and mononuclear pleocytosis. The CSF protein is mildly elevated and glucose levels are normal. Which one of the following is the most likely diagnosis?

- ☐ **A** Herpes simplex encephalitis
- ☐ **B** Cerebral malaria
- ☐ **C** Alcohol withdrawal and alcohol fit
- ☐ **D** Brain abscess
- ☐ **E** Pneumococcal meningitis

272 A 45-year-old man has complained of low back pain of six months' duration. The pain initially radiated to the right leg but two months later he experienced similar pain in the left leg. Which one of the following physical findings is not characteristic of cauda equina syndrome?

- [ ] **A** Significant post-void residual urine volume
- [ ] **B** Positive Babinski sign
- [ ] **C** Perineal anaesthesia
- [ ] **D** Poor anal sphincter tone
- [ ] **E** Absent ankle jerk

273 A 27-year-old man has been admitted with a chest infection. He states that he smokes £30 worth of heroin daily and is asking for methadone to alleviate his subjectively severe withdrawal symptoms. There is no documented evidence that he is an addict and you are cautious about giving him an opiate. The presence of each of the following would support his claim of opiate withdrawal, except

- [ ] **A** Lactorrhoea
- [ ] **B** Mydriasis
- [ ] **C** Panic attacks
- [ ] **D** Piloerection
- [ ] **E** Yawning

274 You have been asked to review a 45-year-old nurse with gross truncal obesity, moon face and abdominal striae. Apparently she has noticed spontaneous leakage of milk from her breasts. The past medical history revealed a previous antidepressant overdose. She drinks two bottles of wine most weekends and has smoked 20 cigarettes a day for the last 20 years. The most likely cause of this patient's cushingoid features is

- [ ] **A** Carcinoma of bronchus with ectopic ACTH
- [ ] **B** Pituitary adenoma
- [ ] **C** Adrenal adenocarcinoma
- [ ] **D** Surreptitious steroid ingestion
- [ ] **E** Chronic alcoholism

275 A 25-year-old man developed a group of itchy blisters on the back and on the extensor surfaces of the limbs. Further tests confirmed the diagnosis of coeliac disease. The patient was prescribed dapsone to ease the skin complaints. Over the next 48 hours the patient experienced improvement in the itching but he noticed that he was passing red-coloured urine. The full blood count showed a haemoglobin of 6 g/dl. Which one of the following is the most appropriate test at this stage?

☐ A Myoglobin concentration in urine
☐ B Haemoglobin levels in urine
☐ C Glucose-6-phosphate dehydrogenase (G6PD) concentration
☐ D Red blood cell osmotic fragility test
☐ E Haemoglobin electrophoresis

276 You have been asked to review a 70-year-old man who was referred because of persistent pain in both knees. He is known to have osteoarthritis of both knees and was recently diagnosed with angina and hypertension. He was taking bendroflumethiazide (bendrofluazide) tablets, paracetamol and codeine. You added a cyclo-oxygenase (COX-2) inhibitor, rofecoxib 25 mg daily, on a regular basis. Your choice of a COX-2 inhibitor is based mostly on the fact that

☐ A It is superior in efficacy compared to other standard non-steroidal anti-inflammatory drugs (NSAIDs)
☑ B It causes fewer gastrointestinal side effects than the standard NSAIDs
☐ C It has the advantage of strong anti-platelet effects and therefore there is no need to add aspirin for patients requiring prevention of ischaemic heart disease
☐ D There is no need to adjust the antihypertensive dosage as it does not cause fluid retention
☑ E It has no effect on the kidneys and it is safe to continue the drug even if the renal function is moderately impaired

277 A 60-year-old farmer, known to have rheumatoid arthritis and hypertension, presents with increasing shortness of breath over the previous three days. He had been resting in bed due to a flare-up of his arthritis. The arterial blood gases reveal: PaO_2 8 kPa, $PaCO_2$ of 4.5 kPa, and pH 7.48. This patient's clinical presentation could be due to each of the following conditions, except

- **A** Fibrosing alveolitis
- **B** Acute pulmonary oedema
- **C** Acute late-onset asthma
- **D** Pulmonary embolism
- **E** Hyperventilation

278 You are asked to see a 45-year-old woman who is brought to the Emergency Department after ingestion of 30 tablets of phenobarbital. The patient is drowsy with shallow infrequent respiratory movements. Which one of the following blood gases results is most likely to match the clinical scenario in this particular patient?

- **A** PaO_2 of 11 kPa, $PaCO_2$ of 4.5 kPa, pH 7.62
- **B** PaO_2 of 9 kPa, $PaCO_2$ of 7.5 kPa, pH 7.35
- **C** PaO_2 of 9 kPa, $PaCO_2$ of 4.6 kPa, pH 7.40
- **D** PaO_2 of 12 kPa, $PaCO_2$ of 4.5 kPa, pH 7.48
- **E** PaO_2 of 8 kPa, $PaCO_2$ of 8 kPa, pH 7.22

279 You are asked to assess a 41-year-old black African-American woman who has rheumatoid arthritis and has been taking methotrexate for three years. She presents with a left-sided pleural effusion. You aspirate about 500 ml of milky pleural fluid. Further analysis of the fluid showed a high triglyceride concentration. Which one of the following is the most likely cause of this patient's illness?

- **A** Lymphoma
- **B** Sarcoidosis
- **C** Tuberculosis
- **D** Rheumatoid-associated pleural effusion
- **E** *Pneumocystis carinii* pneumonia

280 You are asked to review a 75-year-old man with heart failure. He has been admitted with deep vein thrombosis of the right leg. You start him on anticoagulant therapy. Each of the following clinical findings might prompt you to start long-term anticoagulation therapy, except

☐ **A** Atrial fibrillation
☐ **B** Left ventricular aneurysm
☑ **C** Aortic stenosis
☐ **D** Left ventricular thrombus
☐ **E** History of thromboembolic disease

281 A 45-year-old otherwise healthy homosexual man is concerned that he might be HIV-positive but is not willing to have any HIV serology tests done unless a doctor tells him that he is developing symptoms suggestive of HIV infection. Each of the following mucocutaneous lesions should prompt you to advise him to have the test, except

☐ **A** Lipodystrophy
☐ **B** Oral candidiasis
☐ **C** Pemphigoid
☐ **D** Kaposi's sarcoma
☐ **E** Molluscum contagiosum

282 A 50-year-old woman has been feeling tired for weeks. A complete blood count is performed and she is found to have a haemoglobin of 9 g/dl with a total WBC count of 5.5×10^9/l and platelet count of 165×10^9/l. The microscopic appearance of the peripheral blood smear shows hypersegmented neutrophils. Which one of the following laboratory test findings would you most expect to be present?

☐ **A** Low serum iron levels
☐ **B** Positive antinuclear antibody test
☐ **C** Decreased serum B_{12} levels
☐ **D** Glucose-6-phosphate dehydrogenase (G6DP) deficiency
☐ **E** Positive Coombs' test

283 On assuming the horizontal position after standing for a long period of time, the venous blood will be redistributed more evenly between the leg veins and the thoracic veins. This will immediately result in which one of the following responses?

☐ **A** A decrease in stroke volume
☐ **B** A decrease in cardiac output
☐ **C** An increase in the resistance of the peripheral veins
☐ **D** An increase in the central venous pressure
☐ **E** A decrease in the central venous pressure

284 A 65-year-old woman with a two-year history of itching presents with jaundice and excessive fatigue. The antimitochondrial antibodies are positive. The liver biopsy confirms the diagnosis of primary biliary cirrhosis. You would consider each of the following treatments as an essential part of the of this patient's management, except

☐ **A** Low-dose oral steroid therapy
☐ **B** Ursodeoxycholic acid
☐ **C** Colestyramine
☐ **D** Calcium and vitamin D supplements
☐ **E** Liver transplantation

285 A 40-year-old man with a history of recurrent deep venous thrombosis was investigated for four painless, punched-out ulcers on the scrotum. He is married with two children. He denied extramarital sexual contacts. He could not swallow the anti-viral tablets prescribed because of recurrent and painful mouth ulcers. The most likely diagnosis is

☐ **A** Antiphospholipid syndrome
☐ **B** Syphilis
☐ **C** Herpes simplex virus type 2 infection
☐ **D** Behçet's disease
☐ **E** AIDS

286 A 13-year-old schoolgirl who is known to have facial eczema presents with multiple itchy, yellow, crusted lesions over the face and the fingers. As a child she was investigated for a cardiac murmur which was thought to be benign. A swab and culture of the skin lesion grows group A streptococci. This patient is at higher risk of developing which one of the following disorders?

☐ A Subacute bacterial endocarditis
☐ B Glomerulonephritis
☐ C Rheumatic fever
☐ D Diffuse maculopapular skin rash if given amoxicillin antibiotics
☐ E Meningitis

287 A 35-year-old shopkeeper presents with a one-week history of fever, right upper quadrant pain and nausea. He travels twice a year to Pakistan to buy special items for his shop. On examination he is not jaundiced, the liver is tender to palpation and is 6 cm below the right costal margin. Ultrasound liver scan confirms the presence of a 3 × 3 cm, well-defined oval cavity, with a central hypoechoic area, in the right lobe. Which one of the following tests is most helpful in confirming the diagnosis of amoebic liver abscess?

☐ A Serology
☐ B Needle aspiration of the cavity
☐ C Sigmoidoscopy
☐ D Computed tomography of the liver
☐ E Stool microscopy

288 A 45-year-old woman with a 25-year history of diabetes mellitus was referred for further evaluation of three episodes of dysarthria, vertigo and diplopia in the last three months. Each episode lasted for one hour and she was symptom-free between these attacks. Full neurological assessment revealed no neurological deficit. Which one of the following laboratory test findings would be least helpful in the management of this patient?

☐ A Carotid Doppler ultrasound
☐ B Magnetic resonance imaging of the brain
☐ C Echocardiogram
☐ D Coagulation screen
☐ E Full blood count

289 An 18-year-old student presents with fever, sore throat and enlarged cervical lymph glands. The peripheral blood shows atypical lymphocytes and the Paul–Bunnell test is positive. Each of the following is a well-recognised complication of this disorder, except

- ☐ **A** Agranulocytosis
- ☐ **B** Transverse myelitis
- ☐ **C** Hepatitis
- ☐ **D** Meningoencephalitis
- ☐ **E** Endocarditis

290 A 42-year-old woman with pruritis, jaundice, xantholasma and a positive antimitochondrial antibody test has a liver biopsy. Which one of the following histopathology reports is typical of this condition?

- ☐ **A** Partial destruction of interlobular bile ducts, surrounded by mononuclear infiltrates
- ☐ **B** Polymorphonuclear leukocytes inside the interlobular bile ducts
- ☐ **C** Periportal plasma cell infiltration; piecemeal necrosis; bridging fibrosis
- ☐ **D** Epithelioid granuloma in the portal and periportal areas
- ☐ **E** Liver cell necrosis; Mallory body infiltration by neutrophils; perivenular distribution of inflammation

291 A 48-year-old woman has a persistently dry mouth despite regular fluid intake. A biopsy of the inner lip is performed and shows mononuclear cell infiltration of the labial salivary glands. Which one of the following serological tests is most likely to be positive?

- ☐ **A** Anti-Ro antibodies
- ☐ **B** Anti-ribonucleoprotein (anti-RNP)
- ☐ **C** Rheumatoid factor
- ☐ **D** Antinuclear antibodies (ANA)
- ☐ **E** Antimitochondrial antibodies

292 A 70-year-old retired teacher was seen with his son in the Outpatient Clinic. His son had noticed his father getting increasingly forgetful. He repeats himself and often fails to recognise close relatives. Finding his way home even after a small trip to the local shop is becoming increasingly difficult. Which one of the following neuropathological findings is most likely to accompany this patient's illness?

- [ ] **A** Anterior horn degeneration
- [ ] **B** Syrinx formation
- [ ] **C** Demyelinating plaques
- [ ] **D** Axonal degeneration
- [ ] **E** Neurofibrillary tangles

293 A 33-year-old intravenous drug abuser is positive for the human immunodeficiency virus. She has experienced pain on swallowing. Upper endoscopy reveals a few raised, creamy-white plaques and several sharply demarcated small areas of shallow ulceration in the mid- to lower oesophagus. Which one of the following is the most likely cause of this problem?

- [ ] **A** Herpes simplex oesophagitis
- [ ] **B** Cytomegalovirus infection of the oesophagus
- [ ] **C** Barrett's oesophagus
- [ ] **D** Oesophageal candidiasis
- [ ] **E** Oesophageal web

294 A 44-year-old female dancer presents with increasing pain with movement of her knees, hips, elbows and shoulders. A year ago she described migratory arthralgia and myalgia, along with chest pain and an irregular heart rate. This was preceded by a ring-like rash on her right leg that subsided over several weeks. Which one of the following risk factors is most likely to have led to this series of events?

- [ ] **A** Photosensitivity
- [ ] **B** Cocaine abuse
- [ ] **C** Repetitive strain injury
- [ ] **D** Tick bite
- [ ] **E** Exposure to HIV-infected body fluids

295 A 30-year-old secretary has short stature and a webbed neck. She has never had menstrual periods. Which one of the following karyotypes is she most likely to have?

- [ ] **A** 46, XY
- [ ] **B** 47, XYY
- [ ] **C** 47, XXX
- [ ] **D** 45, XO
- [ ] **E** 46, XX

296 A 54-year-old man with a long history of diabetes mellitus presents with chest pain that has been present for several days. The cardiac examination reveals a friction rub. Which one of the following laboratory test findings is most likely to be present?

- [ ] **A** Hyperuricaemia
- [ ] **B** High triglyceride levels
- [ ] **C** Hypocalcaemia
- [ ] **D** Hypoglycaemia
- [ ] **E** Elevated serum urea nitrogen

297 A 46-year-old woman, presents with a two-month history of fatigue. Her friend noticed the new onset of jaundice two weeks ago. The patient reports that she had been in a road traffic accident, sustaining a left femoral comminuted fracture, two years ago. She underwent open reduction and internal fixation of the fracture and received four units of packed red blood cells. Liver function tests reveal: AST 115 U/l, ALT 265 U/l, ALP 33 U/l, albumin 33 g/l, total bilirubin 123 µmol/l, direct bilirubin 116 µmol/l. Which one of the following conditions is she most likely to have?

- [ ] **A** Autoimmune haemolytic anaemia
- [ ] **B** Delayed transfusion reaction
- [ ] **C** Hepatitis C infection
- [ ] **D** Gilbert's syndrome
- [ ] **E** Alcoholic liver disease

298 Tumour markers are substances that can often be detected in higher than normal amounts in the blood, urine or body tissues of some patients with certain types of cancer. Which one of the following statements is false?

- [ ] **A** α-Fetoprotein (AFP) is normally produced by a developing fetus
- [ ] **B** Higher levels of CA 19-9 are encountered in breast cancer
- [ ] **C** CA 125 is used in monitoring ovarian cancer recurrence
- [ ] **D** Elevated PSA levels may be found in benign prostatic hyperplasia
- [ ] **E** In liver cirrhosis CA 19-9 and α-fetoprotein (AFP) levels are elevated

299 A 78-year-old woman presents to the Emergency Department following an overdose of paracetamol and amitriptyline. Following successful medical management, you assess her prior to discharge. Which one of the following features, present on assessment, is most likely to indicate risk of completed suicide after discharge?

- [ ] **A** Her age
- [ ] **B** One previous episode of deliberate self-harm by attempted hanging last year
- [ ] **C** Delusions of poverty
- [ ] **D** Living alone
- [ ] **E** Presence of obsessional symptoms

300 Burkitt's lymphoma is usually linked to Epstein–Barr virus. Each of the following tumours are known to be causally related to certain virus infections except

- [ ] **A** Cervical cancer
- [ ] **B** Hepatoma
- [ ] **C** Kaposi's sarcoma
- [ ] **D** Gastric MALT lymphoma
- [ ] **E** Adult T-cell leukaemia

PAPER FOUR QUESTIONS

301 A 73-year-old retired naval officer was brought by the ambulance to the Emergency Department unconscious. His wife said that three days before he had experienced increasing headache and had vomited twice. This morning she noticed gradual deterioration in the level of consciousness. She thinks his illness is probably related to an incident in which he accidentally hit a lamp-post with his head while they were walking the dog two weeks ago. The most appropriate investigation at this stage is

- [x] **A** Computed tomography (CT) brain scan
- [ ] **B** Skull X-rays
- [ ] **C** Magnetic resonance imaging (MRI) of the brain
- [ ] **D** Radionuclide brain scan
- [ ] **E** Positron emission tomographic (PET) study

302 A 56-year-old retired civil servant is admitted with central chest pain which is radiating to the left arm and jaw. The 12-lead ECG shows left bundle branch block. The cardiac enzymes are normal. He has had three similar admissions in the last six months despite optimum treatment. Similar ECG changes were noticed in previous records. The most appropriate investigation at this stage is

- [ ] **A** Exercise tolerance test
- [ ] **B** Dipyridamole-thallium scintigraphy
- [ ] **C** 99 mTc pyrophsphate imaging
- [x] **D** Exercise thallium scintigraphy
- [ ] **E** Multiple gated acquisition (MUGA) scan

303 A 56-year-old woman was celebrating her birthday at a family reception. The next morning she experienced recurrent abdominal cramps and diarrhoea. On physical examination she was febrile, with a temperature of 38°C. The abdomen was soft, but there was some tenderness at the left iliac fossa. The urea was raised at 12 mmol/l with a normal creatinine level. Stool examination grew *Salmonella typhimurium*. The Infection Control Unit acknowledged the admission of her sister and daughter who are similarly affected. They had been at the same reception. Which one of the following statements is true?

- [ ] A Give intravenous fluids and start intravenous gentamicin 80 mg once daily
- [ ] B Arrange computed tomography of the abdomen
- [ ] C Give intravenous fluids and avoid giving any antibiotics
- [ ] D Arrange ultrasound of the kidneys before initiating any therapy
- [ ] E Quinolones are regarded as the drug of choice for this condition

304 A 56-year-old man has had chronic lower back pain for ten years. Three weeks ago he experienced sudden severe pain in the lower back, radiating to the left leg, worse on bending or coughing. He also complained of pins and needles in the left lower limb. Straight leg raising was at 45° on the left and 90° on the right. The left ankle jerk was absent. Radiographs of the lower lumbar region showed reduced intervertebral spaces at L4/5 and L5/S1, with large osteophyte formation. To confirm the diagnosis promptly which one of the following would you now order?

- [ ] A Computed tomography (CT) of the lumbosacral region
- [ ] B Magnetic resonance imaging (MRI) of the lumbosacral region
- [ ] C Isotope bone scan
- [ ] D Nerve conduction studies
- [ ] E Dual-energy X-ray absorptiometry (DEXA) scan

305 Cyclophosphamide infusion was prescribed in repeated courses for a 28-year-old woman with lupus nephritis. There is evidence of relapse of the nephritis and you considered admitting the patient for cyclophosphamide infusion. The patient asked you to clarify again the complications of this therapy. You consider each of the following to be a potential side effect of this therapy, except

- ☐ **A** Bladder carcinoma
- ☐ **B** Pulmonary fibrosis
- ☐ **C** Hepatic fibrosis
- ☐ **D** Haemorrhagic cystitis
- ☐ **E** Irreversible amenorrhoea

306 A 19-year-old university student has a white cell count of 200 × 10⁹/l and a platelet count of 50 × 10⁹/l. The chest X-ray shows a mediastinal mass. The most likely diagnosis is

- ☐ **A** Sarcoidosis
- ☐ **B** Lymphoma
- ☐ **C** Acute lymphoblastic leukaemia (ALL)
- ☐ **D** Waldenström's macroglobulinaemia
- ☐ **E** Chronic lymphatic leukaemia (CLL)

307 A 60-year-old shop assistant who has smoked 20 cigarettes a day since her teens is admitted with bone pain and weight loss. She is at higher risk for having each of the following malignancies, except

- ☐ **A** Carcinoma of the bronchus
- ☐ **B** Carcinoma of the bladder
- ☐ **C** Oesophageal carcinoma
- ☐ **D** Carcinoma of the breast
- ☐ **E** Carcinoma of the oral cavity

308 A 60-year-old woman is being investigated for rapidly increasing abdominal distension. Ascites was confirmed on physical examination. The α-fetoprotein (AFP) level is 200 μg/l (normal range <10–20 μg/l). Which one of the following is the most likely disorder behind this presentation?

☐ **A** Liver cirrhosis
☐ **B** Germ cell ovarian cancer
☐ **C** Adenocarcinoma of the colon
☐ **D** Carcinoma of the head of the pancreas
☐ **E** Medullary carcinoma of the thyroid gland

309 An echocardiogram confirmed the presence of a vegetation on an incompetent aortic valve in a 60-year-old accountant with severe heart failure. Repeated blood cultures were negative. Each of the following organisms could be responsible for this clinical picture, except

☐ **A** *Chlamydia psittaci*
☐ **B** *Coxiella burnetii*
☐ **C** Coxsackie virus A
☐ **D** *Candida albicans*
☐ **E** *Legionella pneumophila*

310 A 30-year-old man is admitted with excessive fatigue and easy bruising. Physical examination reveals pallor but no lymphadenopathy or hepatosplenomegaly. The full blood count shows: haemoglobin 7.8 g/dl, platelet count 40×10^9/l, neutrophil count 1.5×10^9/l. Which one of the following tests would be most helpful in establishing the diagnosis?

☐ **A** Bone marrow aspiration and cytology study
☐ **B** Radionuclide bone scan
☐ **C** Whole body computed tomography scan
☐ **D** Bone marrow biopsy
☐ **E** Coombs' test

311 As part of your work-up for a patient with musculoskeletal abnormalities you organised karyotyping which shows 46, XX, +21. Which one of the following disorders corresponds to this karyotype?

- [ ] **A** Noonan's syndrome
- [ ] **B** Down's syndrome
- [ ] **C** Klinefelter's syndrome
- [ ] **D** Turner's syndrome
- [ ] **E** Bloom's syndrome

312 A 30-year-old man asked to see you because two of his brothers have been diagnosed with familial hypercholesterolaemia. Which one of the following statements about familial hypercholesterolaemia is false?

- [ ] **A** LDL receptors may be defective
- [ ] **B** Serum LDL is elevated from birth
- [ ] **C** Tendon xanthomata are a feature
- [ ] **D** Migratory arthropathy may be a manifestation
- [ ] **E** Heterozygotes are rarely clinically affected

313 A 34-year-old man known to suffer with acute intermittent porphyria was admitted to hospital with a severe neuromuscular disorder. Haematin was given intravenously with rapid improvement in his symptoms. The main mechanism of action of haematin in intermittent porphyria is through

- [ ] **A** Increasing renal clearance of porphobilinogen
- [ ] **B** Inducing liver metabolism of porphyrins
- [ ] **C** Suppression of δ-aminolaevulinic acid (ALA) synthetase activity
- [ ] **D** Blocking the action of porphyrins at the neuromuscular junctions
- [ ] **E** Stimulation of porphobilinogen synthetase activity

314 A 56-year-old man is admitted with increasing dyspnoea on exertion. He smokes two packs of cigarettes daily. He has orthopnoea and paroxysmal nocturnal dyspnoea. He sustained an anterior myocardial infarction three months earlier. Physical examination shows a pulse of 130 bpm which is irregular. The ECG shows evidence of atrial fibrillation and lateral ischaemia. The chest X-rays and the echocardiograph confirm the presence of cardiomegaly, poor left ventricular function and dilated cardiac chambers. Which one of the following medications would not be recommended in this case?

- **A** Flecainide
- **B** Furosemide (frusemide)
- **C** Nitrate
- **D** Angiotensin-converting enzyme inhibitor
- **E** Warfarin

315 A 25-year-old taxi driver underwent internal fixation of the right tibia. He developed an anaphylactic reaction to infusion of blood. Which one of the following disorders is most likely to be associated with this reaction?

- **A** Hyperimmunoglobulinaemia IgE syndrome
- **B** Selective IgA deficiency
- **C** DiGeorge's syndrome
- **D** C1 esterase inhibitors deficiency
- **E** Adenosine deaminase deficiency

316 Which one of the following is regarded as the most important factor in modulating arterial blood pressure?

- **A** Cardiac output
- **B** Peripheral vascular resistance
- **C** Heart rate
- **D** Preload
- **E** Myocardial contractility

317 A 30-year-old man has had pain and stiffness in his lower back for one year. The pain improves with exercise. Physical examination revealed limited movement at the lumbar spine with loss of lumbar lordosis. Which of the following is most likely to be observed on X-rays of the pelvis and lumbosacral spine?

☐ **A** L4/5 disc space narrowing
☐ **B** Osteophyte formation at L2, L3 and L4 vertebrae
☐ **C** Bilateral sacroiliitis
☐ **D** Normal radiographic findings
☐ **E** Spina bifida occulta

318 A 47-year-old man was admitted to the Intensive Care Unit with coma secondary to fulminant pneumococcal meningitis. He has been ventilated for two weeks and trials to wean him off the ventilator were not successful as there was no respiratory movements to maintain spontaneous breathing. He was thought to have brainstem death. The family and carers were informed and ventilatory support discontinued. In order to confirm brainstem death, each of the following reflexes should be identified as absent on more than one occasion, except

☐ **A** Gag reflex
☐ **B** Corneal reflex
☐ **C** Pupillary reflexes
☐ **D** Knee reflex
☐ **E** Vestibulo-ocular reflexes

319 A 32-year-old African-American woman presents with fever, persistent dry cough and facial skin rash. The chest X-ray shows diffuse reticulonodular shadowing. Which one of the following statements concerning the diagnosis of sarcoidosis is true?

☐ **A** The diagnosis is based on serial angiotensin-converting enzyme (ACE) levels
☐ **B** Definitive diagnosis is based on the histology of transbronchial biopsy tissue
☐ **C** Sarcoidosis affects the reticuloendothelial system but not the bone marrow
☐ **D** Normal pulmonary function studies exclude the diagnosis of sarcoidosis
☐ **E** Lymphadenopathy is the most common abnormal finding on chest X-rays

115

320 A 64-year-old man develops pain and swelling in both knees three days after a cardiac bypass operation. He used to have mild discomfort in both knees whenever he walked more than 300 yards. The most likely diagnosis is

- [ ] **A** Pseudogout
- [ ] **B** Gout
- [ ] **C** Septic arthritis
- [ ] **D** Osteoarthritis
- [ ] **E** Rheumatoid arthritis

321 You have been asked to review a 65-year-old left-handed man who was admitted with rapid decline in the level of consciousness. Computed tomography of the brain was reported as normal. You order a magnetic resonance imaging scan to define the brainstem region because you think the patient might have pontine haemorrhage. Clinical manifestations of this lesion include each of the following, except

- [ ] **A** Hyperpyrexia
- [ ] **B** Nystagmus
- [ ] **C** Quadriplegia
- [ ] **D** Receptive dysphasia
- [ ] **E** Pinpoint pupil

322 A 34-year-old nurse was admitted for the evaluation of recurrent attacks of hypoglycaemia with documented low plasma glucose levels. She developed symptoms after five hours of supervised fast. The plasma insulin and the C peptide levels drawn at the time of symptoms are both markedly elevated. Which one of the following is the most appropriate diagnostic test?

- [ ] **A** Measurement of insulin-like growth factor
- [ ] **B** Glucagon stimulation test
- [ ] **C** Superior mesenteric angiography
- [ ] **D** Measurement of insulin antibodies
- [ ] **E** Glucose tolerance test

323 A 34-year-old woman with hyperprolactinaemia presents with amenorrhoea. Which one of the following manifestations is also caused by high prolactin levels?

☐ **A** Acanthosis nigricans
☐ **B** Osteopenia
☐ **C** Hyperpigmentation
☐ **D** Excessive perspiration
☐ **E** Arthritis of the small joints of the hands

324 A 34-year-old woman was investigated for irregular periods which had persisted despite various types of hormone treatment. She was found to have raised prolactin levels. Which one of the following is likely to be responsible for the elevated prolactin levels?

☐ **A** Ovarian failure
☐ **B** Iron deficiency anaemia
☐ **C** Hyperthyroidism
☐ **D** Oral contraceptive pills
☐ **E** Endometriosis

325 A 24-year-old man with progressive shortness of breath due long-standing emphysema was admitted for further assessment. If an arterial blood gas analysis was performed on the patient while breathing room air, which one of the following results would be most likely?

☐ **A** pH 7.45, $Paco_2$ 6.0 kPa, bicarbonate 15 mmol/l
☐ **B** pH 7.34, $Paco_2$ 10.0 kPa, bicarbonate 36 mmol/l
☐ **C** pH 7.60, $Paco_2$ 3.0 kPa, bicarbonate 17 mmol/l
☐ **D** pH 7.20, $Paco_2$ 3.0 kPa, bicarbonate 8 mmol/l
☐ **E** pH 7.30, $Paco_2$ 8.0 kPa, bicarbonate 26 mmol/l

326 In a healthy 60-year-old man which one of the following is true about water distribution in his body?

☐ A The total body water volume is 12 litres
☐ B The extracellular fluid volume is 6 litres
☐ C The intracellular fluid volume is 10 litres
☐ D The interstitial fluid volume is 5 litres
☐ E The plasma volume is 3 litres

327 A 40-year-old man is admitted with fever and shortness of breath. Physical examination revealed splinter haemorrhages and a cardiac murmur. Echocardiogram identified vegetations. Which one of the following cardiac lesions is the least likely underlying cause of this man's clinical condition?

☐ A Atrial septal defect
☐ B Congenital bicuspid aortic valve
☐ C Patent ductus arteriosus
☐ D Coarctation of the aorta
☐ E Mitral valve prolapse

328 A 45-year-old car mechanic who was investigated for headache and visual disturbance was found to have an anterior pituitary tumour. After surgery histopathology examination of the removed tumour showed abundant acidophils. Which one of the following do anterior pituitary acidophils secrete?

☐ A Growth hormone
☐ B Thyrotrophin-releasing hormone (TRH)
☐ C Follicle-stimulating hormone (FSH)
☐ D Adrenocorticotrophic hormone (ACTH)
☐ E Vasopressin

329 A 45-year-old man presented with a progressive increase in shortness of breath and irregular pulse rate. The on-call doctor suggested a positive inotropic drug. Positive inotropism refers to

- [ ] **A** Decreased stroke volume
- [ ] **B** Movement of ions in relation to chemical gradient
- [ ] **C** Repolarisation of the sinoatrial node
- [ ] **D** Increased conduction velocity
- [ ] **E** Increased contractility of the heart

330 After three weeks in bed following a car accident a 20-year-old student was encouraged by the physiotherapist to do regular exercise. Training exercise such as jogging, swimming and aerobics will have which one of these effects on skeletal muscle tissue?

- [ ] **A** Increase in the number of mitochondria per muscle fibre
- [ ] **B** Increase in the number of nerve fibres per muscle unit
- [ ] **C** Increase in the number of skeletal muscles
- [ ] **D** Increase in the number of motor units
- [ ] **E** Increase in the number of muscle fibres

331 Which one of the following is a cytokine produced by T cells that acts mainly to activate B cells to proliferate?

- [ ] **A** Interferon-γ
- [ ] **B** Interleukin-10
- [ ] **C** Interleukin-2
- [ ] **D** Interleukin-1
- [ ] **E** Interleukin-4

332 The frequency of mutation leading to achondroplasia is influenced by which one of the following?

- [ ] **A** Hot climate
- [ ] **B** Maternal age
- [ ] **C** Paternal age
- [ ] **D** Childhood measles infection
- [ ] **E** Exposure to X-ray radiation

333 You notice that citrate is often used to prevent blood from clotting. Citrate is a useful anticoagulant because of its ability to

- [ ] **A** Chelate calcium
- [ ] **B** Lyse thrombin
- [ ] **C** Block γ-decarboxylation
- [ ] **D** Prevent platelet aggregation
- [ ] **E** Retain fluid and keep blood in a liquid form

334 A patient known to have asthma is telephoned and told that he will have to use the new chlorofluorocarbon- (CFC-) free inhalers as the old CFC-based inhalers are going to be phased out. The recommendation to stop using CFC inhalers was made because of the CFCs ability to

- [ ] **A** Induce bronchogenic carcinoma if inhaled for more than ten years
- [ ] **B** Cause a decrease in the ozone layer
- [ ] **C** Combine with the inhaled drugs and reduce delivery
- [ ] **D** Cause recurrent *Candida* infection of the throat
- [ ] **E** Ignite in the presence of an open oxygen source

335 A previously fit 50-year-old lady was admitted with chest pain of one hour's duration. She has not had any pain since admission six hours ago. The radial pulse was at 80 bpm and regular, blood pressure 120/80 mmHg. Physical examination revealed that cardiac enzymes and ECG were all within normal limits. However, a blood specimen for 'routine' biochemistry reported the following: Na^+ 110 mmol/l, K^+ 2.5 mmol/l, chloride 80 mmol/l, bicarbonate 22 mmol/l, urea 0.02 mmol/l, glucose 50 mmol/l, osmolality 285 mosmol/l. Which one of the following is the most likely diagnosis?

- [ ] **A** Addison's disease
- [ ] **B** Acute myocardial infarction
- [ ] **C** Hypothyroidism
- [ ] **D** Sampling from the 'drip' arm
- [ ] **E** Syndrome of inappropriate antidiuretic hormone secretion (SIADH)

336 A 69-year-old man suffers an acute myocardial infarction (MI). In which one of the following conditions is temporary transvenous pacing most clearly indicated?

☐ **A** Accelerated idioventricular rhythm.
☐ **B** Mobitz type I second-degree atrioventricular (AV) block with normal haemodynamics
☐ **C** Mobitz type II second-degree AV block
☐ **D** First-degree heart block
☐ **E** Bundle branch block known to exist before the acute MI

337 In a population study for HLA (human leukocyte antigen) typing, an increased frequency of HLA-D4 was noted. Which one of the following disorders is associated with this HLA type?

☐ **A** Beçhet's disease
☐ **B** Haemochromatosis
☐ **C** Rheumatoid arthritis
☐ **D** Narcolepsy
☐ **E** Ankylosing spondylitis

338 Which one of the following electrolytes/substances has higher intracellular concentration than extracellular concentration?

☐ **A** Na^+
☐ **B** K^+
☐ **C** Ca^{2+}
☐ **D** Chloride
☐ **E** Bicarbonate

339 A 44-year-old labourer sustained an injury to the left arm. He noticed difficulty in using that arm. Which one of the following features would you expect if the patient has ulnar nerve injury at the elbow?

☐ **A** Varus deformity at the elbow
☐ **B** Typical claw-hand deformity
☐ **C** Absent supinator reflex
☐ **D** Wasting of the thenar eminence
☐ **E** Sensory loss over the thumb

340 A right carotid bruit in an asymptomatic 30-year-old police officer is noted during an annual medical examination. He is physically fit and has no personal or family history of cardiovascular or cerebrovascular disease. Blood tests, including fasting lipid profile, are normal. Further management is probably best done by

- ☐ **A** Carotid magnetic resonance angiography
- ☐ **B** Annual review of the patient
- ☐ **C** Carotid Doppler studies
- ☐ **D** Carotid angiography
- ☐ **E** Recommending no further follow-up

341 A 64-year-old man with poorly controlled hypertension was treated with angiotensin-converting enzyme (ACE) inhibitors. Two months later his blood pressure is well controlled but he reports a troublesome type of cough that is persistent and very irritating. You explain to him that this cough is most likely caused by the ACE inhibitors. Which one of the following statements about the cough associated with ACE inhibitors is true?

- ☐ **A** It is more likely to occur when treating hypertension
- ☐ **B** It is likely to improve on changing to a different ACE inhibitor
- ☐ **C** It is more common in patients who smoke cigarettes
- ☑ **D** It is more common in women than in men
- ☐ **E** It is dose-dependent

342 A 44-year-old man presented with epistaxis and was found to have high blood pressure. Further tests confirmed the diagnosis of polycythaemia rubra vera (PRV). Which one of the following statements about PRV is true?

- ☐ **A** Generalised lymphadenopathy is seen in more than 50% of cases
- ☐ **B** The haemoglobin concentration is elevated but the platelet count is typically low
- ☐ **C** The ESR is characteristically raised
- ☐ **D** The serum erythropoietin is low
- ☐ **E** The serum B_{12} level is low and three-monthly injections of hydroxocobalamin are often necessary

343 **A 58-year-old woman with megaloblastic anaemia attends your clinic. Which one of the following statements about intrinsic factor is true?**

☐ **A** It is a polysaccharide
☐ **B** It is produced by glandular cells in the pancreas
☐ **C** It acts in the terminal ileum
☐ **D** It is important in the absorption of folic acid
☐ **E** Deficiency can be treated with oral vitamin B_{12}

344 **A 64-year-old man is referred because of increasing ankle swelling and shortness of breath. He has rheumatoid arthritis and has been on methotrexate and a small dose steroid for the last nine years. The 24-hour urine protein test shows an albumin concentration of 8 g/l. Kidney biopsy confirms the diagnosis of amyloidosis. Which one of the following statements about amyloid/amyloidosis is true?**

☐ **A** It appears as extracellular basophilic hyaline material
☐ **B** Methotrexate therapy is the most likely cause of amyloidosis in this patient
☐ **C** It shows an apple-green birefringence in fluorescent light
☐ **D** The amyloid protein type is amyloid light chain (AL)
☐ **E** Oral cavity examination often identifies an enlarged tongue

345 **Leptin is a hormone produced in body fat. When injected it is expected to cause which one of the following effects on body function and composition?**

☐ **A** Reduces body fat
☐ **B** Decreases resting energy expenditure
☐ **C** Stimulates production of neuropeptide Y
☐ **D** Increases the feeling of hunger
☐ **E** Acts by stimulating pancreatic lipases

346 A 44-year-old chronic alcoholic woman presents with melaena, jaundice and ascites. She denies chest pain, shortness of breath or cough. The ward nurse informs you that the oxygen saturation is 89% on air. The pulse oximeter may read inaccurately in which one of the following?

- ☐ A Jaundice
- ☐ B Anaemia
- ☐ C Younger patients
- ☐ D Black patients
- ☐ E Hypothermia

347 A 64-year-old retired musician is admitted with shortness of breath. His blood pressure is 80/42 mmHg and the CVP is 16 mmHg. This picture is consistent with a diagnosis of each of the following, except

- ☐ A Tension pneumothorax
- ☐ B Pericardial tamponade
- ☐ C Pulmonary embolism
- ☐ D Congestive cardiac failure
- ☐ E Haemorrhage

348 A 24-year-old man presents to the Emergency Department with a sudden sharp pain in the left side of the chest and shortness of breath. Examination reveals: respiratory rate 40/minute, cyanosis, tracheal deviation to the right and a hyper-resonant left lung. Appropriate treatment includes all the following, except

- ☐ A Intubation and positive-pressure ventilation
- ☐ B Oxygen by mask
- ☐ C Immediate needling of the left side of his chest
- ☐ D Immediate chest X-ray
- ☐ E Estimation of acid–base status

349 You are asked to assess a 21-year-old student who won a county sprinting medal three months ago. Athletes, when resting, differ from normal individuals in having

- [ ] **A** Higher resting cardiac output
- [ ] **B** Higher resting heart rate
- [ ] **C** Decreased muscle mass
- [ ] **D** Lower maximum oxygen consumption
- [ ] **E** Increased muscular efficiency at high blood lactate levels

350 A 35-year-old self-employed builder, married with two children, presented with a five-year history of backache. More recently he had noticed increasing pain in the back radiating to the front of the right thigh. He needed some help to put his trousers on as he could not lift his right leg up. Which one of the following clinical signs would you expect to find on examining this patient?

- [ ] **A** Absent knee tendon jerk
- [ ] **B** Foot-drop
- [ ] **C** Inability to extend the hip
- [ ] **D** Decreased sensation on the dorsum of the foot and big toe
- [ ] **E** Restricted straight leg raising test

351 A group of breast cancer patients were randomised to receive chemotherapy or chemotherapy plus radiotherapy. They were all followed up for a period of 5 years. A chi-square test of the difference in proportions of the two groups alive at 5 years gave a p-value of $p < 0.01$.
Which statement gives the most appropriate interpretation of this result?

- [ ] **A** The difference is very small
- [ ] **B** Less than 1 in 100 patients survived 5 years
- [ ] **C** The two treatments are equally effective
- [ ] **D** The difference is likely to have arisen by chance
- [ ] **E** The difference is statistically significant at the 5% level

352 A 36-year-old man complained of pain in both wrists evolving over eight weeks. He noted swelling around that area but denied stiffness. On examination there was swelling and tenderness just proximal to the wrist joints without limitation of movement. There was also prominent finger clubbing. X-rays revealed periosteal reaction over the lower end of the radius and ulnar. Which one of the following disorders could be the cause of this patient's complaint?

- [ ] A Rheumatoid arthritis
- [ ] B Ankylosing spondylitis
- [ ] C Ulcerative colitis
- [ ] D Diabetes mellitus
- [ ] E Thymoma

353 A 54-year-old woman presents with sudden severe pain and swelling in the left knee. Synovial fluid analysis shows abundant calcium pyrophosphate dihydrate (CPPD) crystals. Which one of the following tests is appropriate for further assessment of this patient's illness?

- [ ] A Creatine kinase
- [ ] B Serum immunoglobulin levels
- [ ] C Thyroid function tests
- [ ] D Antinuclear antibodies
- [ ] E Folic acid levels

354 A 44-year-old bricklayer was working on a fence when a brick fell on his left hand. X-ray of the left hand showed no fracture. During the next four weeks he experienced progressive pain and discomfort in the second and third digits, accompanied by swelling, redness and localised tenderness. The overlying skin is taut and shiny. His temperature, full blood count and ESR were all normal. The most likely diagnosis is

- [ ] A Cellulitis
- [ ] B Acute gout
- [ ] C Reflex sympathetic dystrophy
- [ ] D Rheumatoid arthritis
- [ ] E Dupuytren's contracture

355 A 19-year-old car mechanic was brought by ambulance to the Emergency Department with recurrent tonic–clonic seizures which had been going on for three hours. He failed to regain full consciousness between the seizures. The immediate treatment he should receive is

- [ ] **A** Intravenous phenytoin infusion
- [ ] **B** Intravenous lorazepam
- [ ] **C** Intravenous phenobarbital infusion
- [ ] **D** Intravenous sodium valproate infusion
- [ ] **E** Anaesthesia with thiopentone and ventilation

356 A 24-year-old, otherwise healthy, competitive swimmer presents with severe pain and reduced movement in the right shoulder. He denies any history of trauma. Passive abduction of the shoulder was associated with pain at 60–90°. Sharp pain was also experienced when the patient was asked to drop the arm down to the side of the chest. Shoulder abduction against resistance yielded pain only during the first 35° of movement. All other resisted movements were pain-free. Palpation of the shoulder only produced pain on the superior surface of the greater tubercle of the humerus. The most likely diagnosis is

- [ ] **A** Osteoarthritis of the glenohumeral joint
- [ ] **B** Capsulitis of the shoulder joint
- [ ] **C** Osteoarthritis of the acromioclavicular joint
- [ ] **D** Reflex sympathetic dystrophy
- [ ] **E** Supraspinatus tendonitis

357 A 25-year-old woman presents with inreasing facial hair around the chin and upper lip area. She has also noticed increasing hair growth on the anterior chest. She starts to shave these areas almost every week. She has not had menstrual periods for the last two months. On examination you notice that she has temporal hair recession and a deep voice. The most likely diagnosis is

- [ ] **A** Adrenal carcinoma
- [ ] **B** Polycystic ovarian syndrome
- [ ] **C** Idiopathic hirsutism
- [ ] **D** Minoxidil-induced hirsutism
- [ ] **E** Pregnancy

358 A 55-year-old man presents with weight loss and poor appetite. His wife said that since he was made redundant he has become very difficult to live with as he gets angry very easily and feels guilty about many issues past and present. He stopped playing badminton and rarely visits his friends. Physical examination was unremarkable apart from a documented 8 kg weight loss in the last four months. He was prescribed antidepresssant medication. Each of the following statements is true, except

- [ ] **A** He should feel better in one to three months
- [ ] **B** Patients who respond should be treated for 6–12 months
- [ ] **C** Suicide risk may increase early after using antidepressant
- [ ] **D** Psychomotor retardation responds well to fluoxetine
- [ ] **E** Venlafaxine works best in patients with loss of appetite as the main feature

359 A 33-year-old woman has been noticing that she seems tired and listless. She has had no major illnesses, but reports three bad episodes of 'flu' in the past year which kept her off work for a couple of weeks each time. Laboratory findings include: antinuclear antibody (ANA) positive at 1:1024 with a speckled pattern, no detectable double-stranded DNA antibody, rheumatoid factor negative and RNP antibodies detected at 320 units. The serum creatine kinase is elevated. Her serum urea nitrogen is normal. Which one of the following conditions is she most likely to have?

- [ ] **A** Systemic lupus erythematosus (SLE)
- [ ] **B** Dermatomyositis
- [ ] **C** Mixed connective tissue disease
- [ ] **D** Scleroderma
- [ ] **E** Sjögren's syndrome

360 A 24-year-old national football player collapsed during a match. He was pronounced dead soon after he collapsed. He was born a healthy baby and never had any illness in his life. His last medical review done six months earlier was normal, apart from tall R waves in the lateral chest leads. He had played football since he was 14. The most likely cause of death is

  ☐ **A** Hypertrophic cardiomyopathy
  ☐ **B** Long QT syndrome
  ☐ **C** Aortic stenosis
  ☐ **D** Congenital coronary artery anomalies
  ☐ **E** Arrhythmogenic right ventricular cardiomyopathy

361 A 34-year-old man is referred for an urgent medical opinion. He has been very agitated and has been treated with high doses of antipsychotics. The referring psychiatrist describes a number of clinical features, which are suggestive of neuroleptic malignant syndrome. Which one of the following features is least compatible with this diagnosis?

  ☐ **A** Rigidity
  ☐ **B** Mutism
  ☐ **C** Hyperpyrexia
  ☐ **D** Incontinence
  ☐ **E** Bradycardia

362 The cerebrospinal fluid (CSF) analysis from a 20-year-old butcher suspected of having meningitis shows elevated protein levels and a WCC of 400 cells C/mm³, 90% lymphocytes. Which one of the following organisms is the least likely cause?

  ☐ **A** *Listeria monocytogenes*
  ☐ **B** *Mycoplasma pneumoniae*
  ☐ **C** *Haemophilus influenzae*
  ☐ **D** *Borrelia burgdorferi*
  ☐ **E** *Mycobacterium tuberculosis*

363 A 62-year-old female patient is acting bizarrely on the ward. After assessing her you believe she is not acutely confused but is psychotic. The presence of which one of the following features would provide evidence that the patient is acutely psychotic?

☐ **A** Disorientation
☐ **B** Hypnogogic hallucinations
☐ **C** Echopraxia
☐ **D** Gustatory hallucinations
☐ **E** Tardive dyskinesia

364 A 60-year-old bus driver presented with fever and a sore throat. The full blood count showed evidence of pancytopenia. He is on four different medications but does not carry a list of their names. Pancytopenia is a recognised side effect of each of the following drugs, except

☐ **A** Phenylbutazone
☐ **B** Chloramphenicol
☐ **C** Gold injection
☐ **D** Sulfasalazine
☐ **E** Clindamycin

365 A 44-year-old man is being investigated for a rapid decline in cognitive function and abnormal behaviour. A magnetic resonance imaging (MRI) brain scan is ordered. Each of the following conditions can present with psychiatric symptoms and are associated with abnormalities on MRI brain scanning except

☐ **A** Munchausen's syndrome
☐ **B** Huntington's disease
☐ **C** Depression
☐ **D** Pick's disease
☐ **E** Schizophrenia

366 A 19-year-old man attends with his carer and is presenting with dyspnoea. The carer explains that the patient has learning difficulties, but is unsure of the exact cause. Which one of the following would support a diagnosis of Fragile X syndrome?

- [ ] **A** Absence of secondary male sexual characteristics
- [ ] **B** Micro-orchidism
- [ ] **C** Micrognathism
- [ ] **D** Single palmar crease
- [ ] **E** Strabismus

367 A 40-year-old woman is referred for initiating treatment for depression. She tells you that she suffers from an endocrine disease and is regularly followed-up by the Endocrine Unit. Which one of the following endocrine disorders is least associated with depression?

- [ ] **A** Addison's disease
- [ ] **B** Cushing's syndrome
- [ ] **C** Hyperparathyroidism
- [ ] **D** Hyperthyroidism
- [ ] **E** Hypothyroidism

368 A 35-year-old company director is hospitalised following acute appendicitis. Surgery was uneventful and recovery was going smoothly till the third postoperative day, when he rapidly became confused and fearful, and reported visual and tactile hallucinations of snakes and scorpions crawling over the bedclothes. Physical examination revealed dilated pupils, coarse tremor of the hands and eyelids, profuse sweating, and a rapid, pounding heartbeat. His oral temperature was 37.8°C. His previous medical history was unremarkable. He is described as a moderate social drinker and denied the use of other drugs. The diagnosis most strongly suggested by this description is

- [ ] **A** Septicaemia
- [ ] **B** Post-anaesthesia delirium
- [ ] **C** Alcohol withdrawal delirium
- [ ] **D** Subdural haematoma
- [ ] **E** Uraemia

369 A 22-year-old student was started on chlorpromazine for recently confirmed schizophrenia. The antipsychotic properties of neuroleptic drugs are due to their ability to block which one of the following receptors?

☐ **A** GABAergic
☐ **B** Cholinergic
☐ **C** Dopamine D_2
☐ **D** α-Adrenergic
☐ **E** β-Adrenergic

370 A 23-year-old man is brought to the Emergency Department because of abnormal facial expressions. His mother said that last night he was vomiting and the on-call doctor prescribed metoclopromide tablets. Early this morning he started to experience uncontrolled turning of the head to the left side, his eyes rolling up towards the ceiling and his tongue was involuntarily protruding outside his mouth. These manifestations are intermittent and this last episode has lasted for the past hour. Which one of the following is the most appropriate treatment?

☐ **A** Haloperidol 5 mg intravenously
☐ **B** Benzatropine 2 mg intravenously or intramuscularly
☐ **C** Diazepam 10 mg rectally
☐ **D** Phenytoin 100 mg intravenously
☐ **E** Thiopentone anaesthesia and short-term ventilation

371 A 25-year-old woman presents with a sore mouth. She has not been able to eat for the last three days. Examination of the mouth reveals multiple small round ulcers with a yellow-grey centre surrounded by a red halo over the inner side of the cheeks and roof of the mouth. Which one of the following tests is least likely to be helpful in identifying the cause of these ulcers?

☐ **A** Pathergy skin test
☐ **B** Sigmoidoscopy
☐ **C** Anti-endomysial antibodies
☐ **D** Antinuclear antibodies
☐ **E** Tuberculin skin test

372 A 60-year-old woman who has smoked a pack of cigarettes daily for 40 years is admitted with cough and haemoptysis. Her chest X-rays show a large cavitating mass close to the right hilum. The serum calcium levels are high, as is the parathyroid hormone-related peptide (PTHrP) level. Bronchoscopy and biopsy confirm the diagnosis of carcinoma of the bronchus. Based on the above information, the histopathology of the tumour is most likely to be

- [ ] **A** Adenocarcinoma
- [ ] **B** Small-cell carcinoma
- [ ] **C** Squamous cell carcinoma
- [ ] **D** Fibrosarcoma
- [ ] **E** Alveolar-cell carcinoma

373 A 23-year-old woman is rushed to the Emergency Department with severe asthma. On assessing her, each of the following is included among signs of a severe asthmatic attack except

- [ ] **A** $Paco_2$ of 8 kPa
- [ ] **B** Cyanosis
- [ ] **C** FEV_1 of 0.9 litre
- [ ] **D** Blood eosinophilia
- [ ] **E** Pulsus paradoxicus of 40 mmHg

374 A 56-year-old woman with diffuse systemic sclerosis is referred for further assessment. She reported shortness of breath after minimal exertion and non-productive cough. On examination there was clubbing of the fingers. Auscultation of the chest reveals fine crepitations in the mid- and lower zones. Each of the following blood gas and pulmonary function test abnormalities is typical of this disorder, except

- [ ] **A** Resting $Paco_2$ of 8 kPa
- [ ] **B** Pao_2 of 8 kPa, falling to 6 kPa on minimal exercise
- [ ] **C** FEV_1/FVC ratio of 90% (predicted: 75%)
- [ ] **D** Total lung capacity of 4.8 litres (predicted: 6.5 litres)
- [ ] **E** Diffusion capacity of 15 units (predicted: 25 units)

375 A 33-year-old primiparous woman is two days post-partum, having delivered a normal baby boy. She has become increasingly anxious and has told the midwife she thinks the baby is a 'a changeling'. Careful evaluation fails to identify other bizarre beliefs, and she is continuing to care for the baby. Which one of the following features below is most likely to reassure you the patient is not psychotic?

- [ ] A Absence of auditory hallucinations
- [ ] B The patient says the thoughts are stupid and tries not to think of them
- [ ] C The patient does not believe the thoughts to be hers
- [ ] D The phenomenon is intermittent
- [ ] E The patient has symptoms of anxiety

376 A 39-year-old carpenter presents with rapidly progressive dyspnoea, cough and right-sided chest pain. The plain X-rays of the chest reveal a small, unilateral pleural effusion. Which one of the following disorders is the least likely cause of this patient's illness?

- [ ] A Pulmonary infarct
- [ ] B *Pneumocystis carinii* pneumonia
- [ ] C *Mycoplasma pneumoniae* pneumonia
- [ ] D *Streptococcus pneumoniae* pneumonia
- [ ] E *Coccidioides immitis* pneumonia

377 A 34-year-old woman who has two brothers with Becker's muscular dystrophy came to you asking for further clarification about the chances of her children acquiring the same disease. She has four sons and four daughters. Her husband's family have no history of Becker's muscular dystrophy. Which one of the following statements is true?

- [ ] A All the sons will be normal
- [ ] B All the sons will be carriers
- [ ] C Half the sons will be affected
- [ ] D All the daughters will be carriers
- [ ] E Half the daughters will be affected

378 A 56-year-old man appears to be confused, according to nursing staff. You assess him and find the gentleman to be disorientated to time. Which one of the following diagnoses would be compatible with this finding?

☐ **A** Acute schizophrenia
☐ **B** Anxiety neurosis
☐ **C** Obsessive compulsive neurosis
☐ **D** Korsakoff's psychosis
☐ **E** Manic-depressive psychosis

379 The cerebrospinal fluid (CSF) analysis from a 22-year-old university student suspected to have meningitis shows elevated protein levels, a WCC of 500 cells/mm³, (90% lymphocytes) and a normal glucose concentration. Which one of the following organisms is the most likely cause?

☐ **A** *Streptococcus pneumoniae*
☐ **B** *Neisseria meningitidis*
☐ **C** *Haemophilus influenzae*
☐ **D** *Mycobacterium tuberculosis*
☐ **E** Mumps virus

380 A 48-year-old hairdresser has been troubled with an altered bowel habit and abdominal discomfort for five months. She was told that she has irritable bowel syndrome and that no further investigation is deemed necessary. The development of which one of the following symptoms warrants further evaluation?

☐ **A** Recent onset of nausea
☐ **B** Diarrhoea with mucus discharge
☐ **C** Persistence of symptoms for 24 weeks
☐ **D** Abdominal pain relieved with defaecation
☐ **E** Weight loss

381 The gastroscopy report confirmed the diagnosis of duodenal ulcer in a 40-year-old man. The possibility of *Helicobacter pylori* infection was raised. Which one of the following tests is considered the gold standard for detection of *H. pylori* infection?

☐ A Rapid urease test
☐ B Gastric biopsy histopathology
☐ C Gastric biopsy specimen culture
☐ D Urea breath test
☐ E *H. pylori* IgG antibodies in serum

382 A 63-year-old man underwent gastroscopy for investigation of long-standing history of heartburn and dyspepsia. Barrett's oesophagus was diagnosed. Which one of the following statements about this condition is true?

☐ A It is asymptomatic in most cases
☐ B Approximately 20% per year progress to adenocarcinoma
☐ C It has autosomal recessive inheritance
☐ D *Helicobacter pylori* eradication therapy is very effective initial treatment
☐ E The lesion is usually located at the mid-point of the oesophagus

383 An 80-year-old woman is referred because of severe pain in the mid-thoracic region. Spine X-rays showed wedge fractures of three thoracic vertebrae secondary to osteoporosis. Calcitonin was prescribed. Each of the following statements about calcitonin is true, except

☐ A A rise in calcium level stimulates its release
☐ B It has an analgesic effect
☐ C It is secreted by special cells in the parathyroid gland
☐ D It cannot be given by mouth
☐ E It has anti-resorptive properties

384　A 60-year-old woman was seen at the Fracture Clinic with a wrist fracture following a minor fall. The dual energy X-ray absorptiometry (DEXA) scan showed the T-score in the hip at −2.9 SD and in the spine at −2.7 SD. In addition to adequate doses of vitamin D and calcium, which group of medications is considered the least effective in the treatment of this patient?

- [ ] **A** Calcitonin
- [ ] **B** Bisphosphonates
- [ ] **C** Fluoride
- [ ] **D** Oestrogen
- [ ] **E** Selective oestrogen-receptor modulators (SERMs)

385　A 67-year-old man with end-stage chronic obstructive pulmonary disease (COPD) was admitted to the hospital because of severe respiratory distress. His condition did not improve despite optimum medical therapy. Each of the following parameters is an indication for non-invasive ventilation, except

- [ ] **A** $Paco_2 > 6$ kPa
- [ ] **B** pH of 7.20
- [ ] **C** Respiratory arrest
- [ ] **D** Respiratory rate of 30/minute
- [ ] **E** Accessory muscle use

386　A 30-year-old woman received a liver allograft three months ago. She presented with a two-week history of dysphagia and pain on swallowing. Further tests confirm the diagnosis of cytomegalovirus (CMV) oesophagitis. This patient is at higher risk of developing any of the CMV infections listed below, except

- [ ] **A** Hepatitis
- [ ] **B** Colitis
- [ ] **C** Retinitis
- [ ] **D** Pneumonitis
- [ ] **E** Meningitis

387 A 35-year-old married nurse who works on the Infectious Diseases Unit is exposed to needlestick injury from a needle used to draw blood from a patient known to be HIV-positive. After washing the injury site with soap and water the nurse should be informed of the following facts – which one of the following is false?

- [ ] A The risk of occupational needlestick HIV transmission is lower than for hepatitis C and hepatitis B infections
- [ ] B She should be encouraged to undergo baseline HIV testing
- [ ] C Zidovudine therapy should be initiated if there is any evidence of seroconversion
- [ ] D She should have a further HIV test six months after exposure
- [ ] E She should practice protected sex

388 The histopathology report for a renal biopsy confirms the diagnosis of membranous glomerulonephritis in a 45-year-old black African lady who is known to have nephrotic syndrome. Which one of the following disorders is the least likely to be responsible for this patient's illness?

- [ ] A Diabetes mellitus
- [ ] B Hodgkin's disease
- [ ] C Hepatitis B infection
- [ ] D Systemic lupus erythematosus
- [ ] E Malaria

389 A 54-year-old shop assistant who takes hormone replacement therapy for hot flushes presents with a right deep vein thrombosis (DVT). She is an ex-smoker and obese. She attends the local gym and denies any history of trauma or medical illness. The following elements of the history represent risk factors for DVT in this patient, except

- [ ] A Female gender
- [ ] B Obesity
- [ ] C Smoking history
- [ ] D Age over 50
- [ ] E Oestrogen therapy

390 A 54-year-old divorced teacher who lives alone is seen six weeks after his second myocardial infarction. He has a history of hypercholesterolaemia and diabetes. Current medication includes simvastatin, omeprazole, amlodipine, digoxin, warfarin and glibenclamide. He is currently awaiting further coronary angiography. On examination he has a pulse of 92 bpm (irregular) and evidence of biventricular failure. An ECG shows atrial fibrillation. He is depressed with sustained low mood, anhedonia, early morning wakening, poor appetite and weight loss. He says the future is bleak and after your assessment you feel he needs an antidepressant. Which one of the following would be most appropriate?

- [ ] **A** Amitriptyline
- [ ] **B** Citalopram
- [ ] **C** Dothiepin
- [ ] **D** Fluoxetine
- [ ] **E** Venlafaxine

391 A 28-year-old nurse attends the Outpatient Clinic worried about a facial mole that she has had since she was a child. She is a sun lover and enjoys travelling to hot countries. After reading a health magazine she became aware that moles can change into malignant melanoma. Which one of the following features is not considered a high risk factor for the development of malignant melanoma?

- [ ] **A** Facial lesions
- [ ] **B** Bleeding
- [ ] **C** Development of satellite lesions
- [ ] **D** Itching
- [ ] **E** Rapid enlargement in size

392 A 60-year-old man who has been treated for recurrent attacks of acute gout has persistently elevated serum uric acid levels. Treatment with which one of the following drugs would significantly lower the serum uric acid levels?

- [ ] **A** Indometacin
- [ ] **B** Colchicine
- [ ] **C** Prednisolone
- [ ] **D** Allopurinol
- [ ] **E** Low-dose aspirin

393 A 64-year-old man has had chronic pain and discomfort in his right knee for many years. He uses a stick to help him walk. X-ray of the knee joint shows evidence of moderately severe osteoarthritis. Which one of the following statements is true?

☐ A He should hold the stick in the left hand
☐ B The right knee will demonstrate a valgus (knocked-knee) deformity
☐ C Chronic knee arthritis is often associated with disuse wasting of the calf muscles
☐ D Aspiration of more than 30 ml of synovial fluid is unusual and goes against the diagnosis of osteoarthritis
☐ E The presence of a Baker's cyst behind the right knee would establish rheumatoid arthritis as the cause of the joint problem

394 A 54-year-old man has had difficulty walking on his left foot for the last year. He has diffuse, non-tender tarsal soft tissue swelling. Neurological examination shows an absent ankle jerk. X-rays of the foot show joint space narrowing with large osteophyte formation, subchondral fractures and loose bodies. Further tests show: urea 7 mmol/l, creatinine 130 μmol/l, glucose 11 mmol/l, rheumatoid factor positive at 1/40, ANA negative and ESR 20 mm/h. The most likely diagnosis is

☐ A Osteoarthritis
☐ B Gouty arthritis
☐ C Rheumatoid arthritis
☐ D Reflex sympathetic dystrophy
☐ E Neuropathic joint disease

395 You are asked to review a 65-year-old right-handed man who was admitted three days earlier with dysphasia and right-sided dense hemiplegia. He is known to have hypertension. Computed tomography of the brain showed haemorrhage in the left fronto-parietal area. He has been comatose for the last 24 hours and has a conjugate gaze palsy. The radial pulse is 55 bpm and the blood pressure is 178/118 mmHg. You consider that each of the following features are associated with poor functional recovery from stroke in this patient, except

- [ ] **A** Conjugate gaze palsy
- [ ] **B** Haemorrhagic stroke
- [ ] **C** Right-sided hemiplegia
- [ ] **D** Prolonged coma
- [ ] **E** Hypertension

396 A 38-year-old woman has Leber's hereditary optic atrophy (a mitochondrial chromosome disorder). What proportion of her son's children will be affected with the disease and what proportion of her daughter's children will be affected with the disease?

- [ ] **A** Son's children 25%; daughter's children 75%
- [ ] **B** Son's children 0%; daughter's children 100%
- [ ] **C** Son's children 50%; daughter's children 50%
- [ ] **D** Son's children 75%; daughter's children 25%
- [ ] **E** Son's children 100%; daughter's children 0%

397 A 24-year-old woman with systemic lupus erythematosus has developed pain in the right groin. She has been limping for the last three weeks and has had to use a stick in order to walk. She was in hospital with nephritis six months ago. She was treated with prednisolone (40 mg daily) for three months but this was tapered to 5 mg a day over a two-month period with no evidence of exacerbation of her nephritis. On examination there was pain and significant restriction of movement of the right hip. Which one of the following is the most likely cause of the hip pain?

- [ ] **A** Flare-up of lupus arthropathy
- [ ] **B** Septic arthritis
- [ ] **C** Osteoarthritis
- [ ] **D** Femoral vein thrombosis
- [ ] **E** Osteonecrosis

398 An 85-year-old woman with long-standing generalised muscle aches and pain, fatigue and depression is told she either has fibromyalgia or polymyalgia rheumatica (PMR). Her erythrocyte sedimentation rate (ESR) came back at 75 mm/hour. Which one of the following statements is true?

☐ A The raised ESR rules out fibromyalgia as a possible diagnosis
☐ B A normal ESR excludes PMR
☐ C Non-steroidal anti-inflammatory drugs (NSAIDs) remain the mainstay of treatment for PMR
☐ D Both conditions might predispose to giant cell arteritis
☐ E Unlike polymyalgia rheumatica, the course of fibromyalgia rarely extends beyond one year

399 The diagnostic ability of a test for the detection of prostate cancer in men aged over 50 years was assessed against a gold standard (assumed to be 100% correct). The sensitivity of the test was determined. Which statement gives the most appropriate description of sensitivity?

☐ A High sensitivity is associated with high specificity
☐ B Sensitivity will decrease as the prevalence of prostate cancer in the population decreases
☐ C Sensitivity can be calculated from data on just those subjects having the gold standard diagnosis of prostate cancer
☐ D If the sensitivity is 100% then there would be no false positive results with the test
☐ E Sensitivity = 100% − specificity

400 A 58-year-old man presents with general fatigue, tiredness and excessive itching. Physical examination reveals a blood pressure of 170/100 mmHg and a palpable spleen. The blood report shows a haemoglobin of 18 g/dl and white cell count of 16 × 10⁹/l. The most appropriate test at this stage is

☐ A Bone marrow aspiration and trephine biopsy
☐ B Whole body computed tomography
☐ C Ultrasound examination of the liver
☐ D Red cell mass
☐ E Serum protein electrophoresis

Answers

PAPER ONE ANSWERS

1 B: The patient was given supplemental oxygen in the ambulance
This patient suffers with chronic obstructive pulmonary disease (COPD) with an acute exacerbation secondary to a chest infection as evident on the chest X-ray. In this condition one would expect evidence of hypoxia, with low PaO_2 and normal or raised $PaCO_2$. The high PaO_2 is most likely to be due to supplemental high-concentration oxygen received before arrival at the hospital, most probably in the ambulance. We used to believe that the elimination of the hypoxic drive by supplemental oxygen led to hypoventilation and hypercapnia with subsequent impairment of the level of consciousness. More recent data suggest that the major processes which contribute to worsening hypercapnia in patients with COPD when they are given supplemental oxygen are (in order of decreasing importance):

- impaired ventilation–perfusion matching due to attenuation of hypoxic pulmonary vasoconstriction
- decreased binding affinity of haemoglobin for carbon dioxide
- decreased minute ventilation.

2 E: Aortic stenosis
The carotid pulse contour is very similar to that of the central aortic pulse, the delay in the onset of the ascending limb of the carotid pulse compared with the central aortic pulse being only about 20 ms. Examination of the carotid pulse therefore provides the most accurate representation of changes in the central aortic pulse. The arterial pulse in aortic stenosis has been described as 'parvus and tardus', ie it is small or weak and rises slowly. The carotid pulse in aortic stenosis is usually slow in upstroke and diminished in amplitude (parvus and tardus) reflecting the delay in outflow throughout systole. In contrast to aortic stenosis, the initial upstroke is typically brisk in patients with HOCM, in whom obstruction develops in mid-systole. A 'spike and dome' pulse is the name given to the carotid pulse in HOCM. Corrigan's (or waterhammer pulse) is characterised by an abrupt, very rapid upstroke of the peripheral pulse (percussion wave), followed by rapid collapse. It is best appreciated by raising the arm abruptly and feeling for the characteristics in the radial pulse. Corrigan's pulse probably results from very rapid ejection of a large left ventricular stroke volume into a low-resistance arterial system. It therefore occurs most commonly in chronic, haemodynamically significant aortic regurgitation. Dissecting aneurysm is associated with absent, delayed or unequal peripheral pulses. Alcoholic

cardiomyopathy is not associated with a characteristic wave pulse *per se*. However, when it causes left ventricular failure and mitral regurgitation it might manifest with pulsus alternans.

3 C: Rheumatoid arthritis

Acute gout is intensely inflammatory, and is therefore characterised by severe pain, redness, swelling, and disability. At least 80% of initial attacks involve a single joint, typically in the lower extremity, most often at the base of the great toe (at the first metatarsophalangeal joint), known as 'podagra', or in the knee. Trauma, surgery, starvation, alcohol ingestion, dietary overindulgence, and ingestion of drugs (eg diuretics, ciclosporin and low-dose aspirin) which affect serum urate concentrations may all promote gouty attacks. Similarly, chronic disorders such as diabetes mellitus, obesity, hyperparathyroidism and hypothyroidism are associated with increased incidence of acute gouty attacks. Rheumatoid arthritis is not associated with increased incidence of hyperuricaemia or gout.

4 C: Poor performance of the serial sevens test

Cognitive problems such as poor concentration, impaired memory, difficulty with word finding, acalculia or spatial disorientation are often part of other psychological conditions. The individual pattern that develops usually reflects the patient's coping mechanisms used to deal with stress or chronic illness, rather than a specific disease process. However, features secondary to neuronal loss represent an organic illness that needs to be positively identified and treated. Visual rather than auditory hallucinations is a feature consistent with an underlying organic disorder. Hemianopia, dysphasia and nystagmus are specific signs of neuronal damage within the brain.

5 E: Incoherence

The symptoms of schizophrenia are classified as either positive or negative. Positive symptoms, like hallucinations and delusions, are outward expressions that usually involve distorted perceptions of reality. Positive symptoms (excesses) also include disorganised speech (implies thought disorder), incoherence and loose associations. Around a half to three-quarters of people with chronic schizophrenia exhibit some features of the negative symptoms of schizophrenia. The four major clinical subgroups of negative symptoms are affective, communicative, conational, and relational.

1. Affective: (blunted affect) – includes deficits in facial expression, eye contact, gestures, and voice pattern. The inability to experience pleasure (anhedonia) and lack of a sense of caring (apathy).

2. Communicative: the patient's speech may be reduced in quantity (poverty of speech) and information (poverty of content of speech). In mild forms of impoverished speech (alogia) the patient makes brief, unelaborated statements; in the more severe form the patient can be virtually mute.
3. Conational: the patient may show a lack of drive or goal-directed behaviour (avolition). They fail to initiate activities, participate grudgingly, and require frequent direction and encouragement.
4. Relational: interest in social activities and relationships is reduced (asociality). Even enjoyable and recreational activities are neglected. Interpersonal relations may be of little interest. Friendships become rare and shallow, with little sharing of intimacy. Contacts with family are neglected. Sexual interest declines. As symptoms progress, patients become increasingly isolated.

6   E: PR-segment depression

In acute pericarditis the ECG typically shows ST-segment elevation in all leads, with an upward concavity of the elevation (the so-called 'smiling face'). The PR segment is depressed but not prolonged. Unlike in myocardial infarction, there is no reciprocal change, and T waves are not peaked or tall.

7   A: α_2-Macroglobulin

Inherited thrombophilia is a genetic tendency to venous thromboembolism. Clinical features suggesting the presence of inherited thrombophilia include:

- Thrombosis at an early age (<45 years)
- A positive family history of thrombosis
- Thrombosis at unusual sites (eg cerebral vein or mesenteric vein)
- Recurrent thrombosis.

This patient satisfies the criteria and should be screened for a possible cause for inherited thrombophilia. Factor V Leiden is the most common cause of the syndrome, accounting for 40–50% of cases. The prothrombin gene mutation, deficiencies in protein S, protein C, or antithrombin (formerly known as antithrombin III) account for most of the remaining cases, while rare causes include plasminogen and heparin cofactor-II deficiencies and dysfibrinogenaemia.

8   E: Multiple endocrine neoplasia syndrome (MEN I)

Multiple endocrine neoplasia (MEN) I is a hereditary disorder in which one, or often two or more of the following glands develop hyperplasia or adenoma (tumour): the parathyroid 80%, the pancreas 70%, the pituitary and, rarely, the adrenals and thyroid gland. It is sometimes called multiple endocrine adenomatosis or Wermer's syndrome, after one of the first doctors to recognise it. Most people affected with this syndrome seek medical treatment because of one of the following: peptic ulcer disease, symptoms related to low blood sugar, symptoms related to high serum calcium levels or kidney stones, or symptoms related to pituitary problems such as headache. Risk factors are a family history of this disorder, a previous pituitary tumour, and a history of Zollinger–Ellison syndrome.

9 E: Tuberculous pleural effusion

Pleural fluid eosinophilia (defined by pleural fluid eosinophils representing more than 10% of the total nucleated cells) usually suggests a benign, self-limited disease, commonly associated with air or blood in the pleural space. However, two more recent studies have found that malignancy was as common in eosinophilic as in non-eosinophilic pleural effusions. The differential diagnosis of pleural fluid eosinophilia includes:

- Pneumothorax
- Haemothorax
- Pulmonary infarction
- Benign asbestos pleural effusion
- Parasitic disease
- Fungal infection (coccidioidomycosis, cryptococcosis, histoplasmosis)
- Drugs
- Malignancy (carcinoma, lymphoma).

Pleural fluid eosinophilia appears to be a rare finding with tuberculous pleurisy on the initial thoracentesis.

10 D: Hypercalcaemia

In hypokalaemia there is depression of the ST segment, a decrease in the amplitude of the T wave, and an increase in the amplitude of U waves (which occur at the end of the T wave). The QT segment is prolonged. Amiodarone, a complex anti-arrhythmic agent with potassium channel blocking activity, causes QT prolongation. Similarly, the QT interval is prolonged in hypomagnesaemia and with diuretic use. Acute myocardial infarction, heart failure, and cardiac hypertrophy are associated with a prolonged QT interval. Hypercalcaemia, however, causes shortening of the QT interval, primarily due to a decrease in ST-segment duration.

11   C: C8

It is agreed that complement deficiency plays an important role in increased susceptibility to meningococcal infection. Deficiency of components of the membrane attack complex (MAC, C5–C9) is associated with infection by *Neisseria* species (meningococcal and gonococcal). The infections, often with unusual serotypes, are rarely fulminant but tend to recur.

12   D: Wegener's granulomatosis

The clinical features are typical of Wegener's granulomatosis. Classic Wegener's granulomatosis is a form of systemic vasculitis that primarily involves the upper and lower respiratory tracts and the kidneys. The most common presenting symptoms include persistent rhinorrhoea, purulent/bloody nasal discharge, oral and/or nasal ulcers, polyarthralgias, myalgias, or sinus pain. Other frequent early complaints relate to the lower respiratory tract and include cough, dyspnoea, haemoptysis (due to an alveolar capillaritis, necrotic lesions or endobronchial disease) and pleuritic pain. Kidney involvement manifests with acute renal failure, urinalysis showing red cells, red-cell and other casts, and proteinuria. Other organ systems that may become involved include joints, eyes, skin, nervous system and the heart.

Tuberculosis is known to cause cavitations in the lungs and might also involve the kidneys. Sometimes it is difficult to differentiate these disorders but upper airways disease and high titres of antineutrophil cytoplasmic antibodies (cANCA) will favour Wegener's granulomatosis. Similarly, carcinoma of the bronchus, which might be associated with lung cavity and glomerulonephritis, is not usually associated with upper airway disease.

Pulmonary lesions in sarcoidosis include bilateral hilar adenopathy and interstitial apical infiltrates; in stage 4 disease there is advanced fibrosis. It rarely causes lung cavitation. Clinically important renal involvement is an occasional problem in sarcoidosis: hypercalciuria and hypercalcaemia are most often responsible, but granulomatous interstitial nephritis or glomerular disease may be seen on rare occasions. The finding of granulomatous inflammation on biopsy of an artery or perivascular area is highly suggestive of Wegener's granulomatosis. Non-caseating granulomata of the lung are typical of sarcoidosis. Pulmonary lesions are most commonly found in the alveolar septa and in the walls of the bronchi.

13 C: Pork

Cysticercosis is a systemic illness caused by dissemination of the larval form of the pork tapeworm, *Taenia solium*. Encystment of larvae can occur in almost any tissue. Involvement of the central nervous system (CNS), known as neurocysticercosis (NCC), is the most clinically important manifestation of the disease.

Humans are the definitive *T. solium* hosts and can carry an intestinal adult tapeworm. Intermittent faecal shedding of egg-containing proglottids or free *T. solium* eggs ensures that the intermediate host (normally pigs) will ingest the excreted eggs in contaminated food or water. *T. solium* embryos penetrate the gastrointestinal mucosa of the pig and are disseminated through the bloodstream to peripheral tissues, resulting in the formation of larval cysts (cysticerci). When undercooked pork is consumed, an intestinal tapeworm will again be formed, completing the life cycle of the worm. Although humans eating pork is a crucial step in completing the life cycle of the parasite, cysticercosis itself develops when humans ingest the eggs of *T. solium (not the pork) and hence man acts as an accidental intermediate host in whom the larval cysts* (cysticerci) may appear in any tissue in the body. Having said that, the eating of contaminated pork is essential in maintaing the life cycle of the parasite and hence promoting the disease's existence. Humans develop *Taenia saginata* tapeworm infection by eating raw or undercooked beef.

14 B: Diclofenac sodium

Aspirin-induced asthma (AIA) is especially common in asthmatics with nasal polyps and sinusitis, with a prevalence of 20–30% in these subjects. AIA was originally thought to be due to an 'allergy' to aspirin; however, it is now clear that most patients also react to structurally distinct non-steroidal anti-inflammatory drugs (NSAIDs), suggesting non-allergic mechanisms are involved in this syndrome. Patients with AIA tend to have more severe asthma than patients without aspirin sensitivity. However, complaints related to nasal polyposis and chronic rhinosinusitis may be more troubling to the patient on a day-to-day basis than recurrent bronchospasm. Diclofenac sodium is a NSAID and therefore its use should be avoided in this patient.

15 E: Haemochromatosis

The clinical presentation is typical of carpal tunnel syndrome. Carpal tunnel syndrome (CTS) is the most common nerve entrapment disorder. It is caused by increased pressure and consequent compression of the median nerve within the anatomic area referred to as the carpal tunnel. Tinel's sign is tested for by tapping over a compressed nerve at the wrist. It is positive if it reproduces pain and paraesthesia, proximal or distal to the site of compression. The test is positive in CTS. All of the above cause CTS except haemochromatosis which does not lead to entrapment of the median nerve at the wrist.

16 D: A 'spike and dome' carotid pulse

The carotid pulse in aortic stenosis is usually slow in upstroke and diminished in amplitude (parvus and tardus) reflecting the delay in outflow throughout systole; in contrast to aortic stenosis, the initial upstroke is typically brisk in patients with HOCM in whom obstruction develops in mid-systole. A slow-rising carotid pulse is typical of aortic stenosis.

A more marked inspiratory decrease in arterial pressure exceeding 20 mmHg is termed 'pulsus paradoxus'. This is easily detectable by palpation, although it should be evaluated with a sphygmomanometer. When the cuff pressure is slowly released, the systolic pressure at expiration is first noted. With further slow deflation of the cuff, the systolic pressure during inspiration can also be detected. The difference between the pressures during expiration and inspiration is the magnitude of the pulsus paradoxus. Pulsus paradoxus is an important physical finding in cardiac tamponade. In addition to tamponade, pulsus paradoxus can occur in chronic obstructive pulmonary disease, hypovolaemic shock, and infrequently in constrictive pericarditis and restrictive cardiomyopathy.

Pulsus bisferiens is characterised by two systolic peaks of the aortic pulse during left ventricular ejection, separated by a mid-systolic dip. Pulsus bisferiens is frequently observed in patients with haemodynamically significant (but not mild) aortic regurgitation. In patients with mixed aortic stenosis and aortic regurgitation, pulsus bisferiens occurs when regurgitation is the predominant lesion.

A dicrotic pulse results from the accentuated diastolic dicrotic wave that follows the dicrotic notch. It tends to occur when the dicrotic notch is low, as in patients with decreased systemic arterial pressure and vascular resistance (eg in fever). A dicrotic pulse also may be present in patients with severe heart failure, hypovolaemic shock, or cardiac tamponade, conditions associated with a decreased stroke volume and elevated systemic vascular resistance.

17 D: Calcium oxalate stones are the most likely cause of the renal colic

More than 80% of calculi in patients with gout are composed entirely of uric acid, with the remainder containing calcium oxalate or calcium phosphate surrounding a central nidus of uric acid. The three major risk factors for uric acid nephrolithiasis are: increased uric acid excretion; reduced urine volume; and a low urine pH, a setting in which most of the uric acid exists as the intact insoluble acid rather than the soluble urate anion.

Antihyperuricaemic therapies such as allopurinol are used in the prevention and reversal of the consequences of urate crystal deposition in joints (gouty arthropathy), urinary tract (nephrolithiasis), renal interstitium (urate nephropathy), and tissue and parenchymal organs (tophi). Oral colchicine (0.6 mg twice daily) is useful in at least some patients with a prior history of gout. Suppression of chemotactic factor release by synovial lining cells appears to underlie the prophylactic action of colchicine.

18 D: Fibrosing alveolitis

Fibrosing alveolitis is almost always an adult disorder, typically occurring in patients over the age of 50, although it can manifest in the elderly patient. It is usually progressive and in most patients it is reported to have been present for more than six months before presentation. On physical examination, crackles are detected on chest auscultation in more than 80% of patients. These are typically 'dry,' end-inspiratory, and 'Velcro' in quality, and are most common in the lung bases. Clubbing is noted in 25–50% of patients.

Physical findings of pulmonary TB are not specific and are usually absent in mild disease. Physical signs of apical cavity pleural thickening or effusion are often encountered in more severe disease. Rales may be present throughout inspiration, or may be heard only after a short cough (post-tussive rales). TB is not associated with clubbing. Although bronchiectasis is associated with clubbing of the fingers, crepitations are often coarse and localised to one segment or lobe. Carcinoma of the bronchus is a possible diagnosis in a heavy smoker who has clubbing of the fingers but it is often associated with physical signs of consolidations, cavities or effusions. Bilateral fine crepitations are not a feature of carcinoma of the bronchus. Clubbing of the fingers is not a feature of chronic obstructive pulmonary disease.

19 A: Haemochromatosis
The clinical manifestations of iron accumulation (haemochromatosis) include liver disease, skin pigmentation, diabetes mellitus, arthropathy, impotence in men, and cardiac enlargement with or without heart failure or conduction defects. The most common presenting symptom is twinges of pain on flexing the small joints of the hand, particularly the second and third metacarpophalangeal (MCP) joints. This is associated with characteristic radiological findings: squared-off bone ends and hook-like osteophytes in the MCP joints, particularly in the second and third MCP joints.

20 E: Leukocyte karyotyping
The signs described are strong evidence of a specific cause for primary hypogonadism, namely Klinefelter's syndrome. Determination of the peripheral leukocyte karyotype should be performed to determine if this syndrome is present. The finding of decreased production of sperm and/or decreased production of testosterone will confirm the diagnosis of hypogonadism. Supranormal serum concentrations of FSH alone or of FSH and LH indicate that the patient has primary hypogonadism. Testicular biopsy does not usually provide more information than the sperm count. MRI of the sellar area should be performed in a man who has acquired (secondary) hypogonadism.

21 A: Fluid restriction
Hyponatraemia with high urine osmolality is characteristic of the syndrome of inappropriate antidiuretic hormone secretion (SIADH). This results from ADH-induced retention of ingested or infused water. Appropriate therapy in this disorder depends on the degree of hyponatraemia and the presence or absence of symptoms. Only patients with symptoms require rapid initial correction: overly rapid correction in any patient should be avoided because it can lead to neurological complications from osmotic demyelination. Water restriction is the mainstay of therapy in asymptomatic hyponatraemia and in chronic SIADH due, for example, to a small cell carcinoma of the lung. The associated negative water balance raises the plasma sodium concentration toward normal. Salt plus a loop diuretic, demeclocycline or lithium should be considered only in the rare patient with persistent, marked hyponatraemia who is unresponsive to, or who cannot tolerate, water restriction.

22 E: Positive Babinski sign

A positive Babinski sign is a hard neurological sign indicating an upper motor neurone lesion. This sign is never encountered in psychiatric disorders. Although many of the other features are probably characteristic of either type of disorder, none of them is exclusive.

23 D: Enalapril therapy

Gynaecomastia is defined histologically as a benign proliferation of the glandular tissue of the male breast, and clinically by the presence of a rubbery or firm mass extending concentrically from the nipple(s). Fat deposition without glandular proliferation is termed pseudogynaecomastia (often seen in obese men).

Causes include: persistent pubertal gynaecomastia, drugs, cirrhosis or malnutrition, primary hypogonadism, testicular tumours, secondary hypogonadism, hyperthyroidism, and chronic renal insufficiency. There is no detectable abnormality in 20% of cases.

There are many drugs that have been associated with gynaecomastia. The pathophysiological mechanism for some, such as oestrogens or anti-androgens, is quite clear. However, for others, such as spironolactone, the mechanisms seem to be more complex. Spironolactone can increase the aromatisation of testosterone to estradiol, enhance the conversion of testosterone to androstenedione, decrease the testosterone production rate by the testes, and displace testosterone from sex-hormone-binding globulins (SHBG), thereby increasing its metabolic clearance rate. Spironolactone also can act as an anti-androgen by binding to androgen receptors and displacing testosterone and dihydrotestosterone from the receptors.

Germ cell tumours account for approximately 95% of testicular neoplasms. Between 2.5% and 6% of affected patients have gynaecomastia at the time of presentation. In adults, large cell carcinoma of the lung, gastric carcinoma, renal cell carcinoma and, occasionally, hepatoma have been associated with gynaecomastia, due to ectopic production of human chorionic gonadotrophin (HCG).

24 C: *Staphylococcus aureus*

Virtually any microbial pathogen is capable of causing bacterial arthritis. *Staphylococcus aureus* is the most common bacterium infecting adult joints.

25 D: Pseudohypoparathyroidism

Children with pseudohypoparathyroidism present with hypocalcaemia and hyperphosphataemia, but PTH levels are elevated, indicative of resistance to all the actions of PTH. Two types of pseudohypoparathyroidism have been described: patients with type 1a disease often have round facies, short stature and short metacarpal and metatarsal bones; patients with the type 1b disease have hypocalcaemia but do not have these phenotypic abnormalities. It has been suggested that PTH resistance is confined to the kidney in the type 1b disorder, leading to hypocalcaemia, hyperphosphataemia and secondary hyperparathyroidism.

26 C: Addison's disease

Addison's disease is an autoimmune disease and often associated with other organ-specific autoimmune disorders such as insulin-dependent diabetes and hypothyroidism. Hyperpigmentation, which is evident in nearly all patients with primary adrenal insufficiency, is the most characteristic physical finding. It is caused by increased melanin content in the skin, due to the melanocyte-stimulating activity of the high plasma ACTH concentrations. The resulting brown hyperpigmentation is generalised, but is most conspicuous in areas exposed to light (such as the face, neck, and backs of the hands), or areas exposed to chronic friction or pressure (such as the elbows, knees, spine, knuckles and waist). Also, patchy pigmentation is seen on the inner surface of lips and the buccal mucosa, along the line of dental occlusion.

Vitiligo is the result of autoimmune destruction of dermal melanocytes and manifests as patchy areas of depigmented skin which occur on the trunk or extremities. ACTH deficiency (panhypopituitarism) does not result in hyperpigmentation.

The characteristic mucocutaneous pigmentations (melanin spots) of Peutz–Jeghers syndrome are present in more than 95% of patients and are caused by the presence of pigment-laden macrophages in the dermis. They are typically flat, blue-grey to brown spots, 1–5 mm in size, that look like freckles and are commonly found on the lips and in the perioral region, on the buccal mucosa (66%), and on the hands and feet.

27 C: Left middle cerebral artery

Middle cerebral artery stroke results in contralateral hemiplegia and hemianasthaesia that is more marked in the upper limb and face, with relative sparing of the leg.

28 E: Sarcoidosis

The presence of objective evidence of dry mouth and/or dry eyes in a patient presenting with sicca symptoms and who is positive for anti-Ro antibodies is highly suggestive of Sjögren's syndrome (SS). This is a chronic inflammatory disorder characterised primarily by diminished lacrimal and salivary gland secretions, resulting in symptoms of dry eyes and dry mouth. SS is characterised by polyclonal B-cell activation and lymphocytic infiltration of the exocrine glands. The risk of non-Hodgkin's lymphoma (NHL) is said to be 44 times higher than in the normal population, with an individual risk of approximately 4–10%. Mild proteinuria and renal tubular dysfunction can occur in SS, resulting in renal tubular acidosis and polyuria due to nephrogenic diabetes insipidus. Hypothyroidism is more common in patients with SS, although the data suggest no true increase in the prevalence of thyroid disease in SS. This observation may be explained by the fact that patients with SS, being older and predominantly female, have a higher incidence of thyroid disease than the general population. Keratoconjunctivitis occurs in up to 5% of patients with sarcoidosis. However, although the same eye abnormalities occur in SS and sarcoidosis, there is no evidence for increased prevalence of sarcoidosis in SS.

29 C: Serum C4 is low

Hereditary angioneurotic oedema is an autosomal dominant inherited condition caused by a deficiency of C1 esterase inhibitor. This results in intermittent episodes of spontaneous complement activation. Clinically, the patient suffers oedema of the skin and mucosal surfaces. Fatalities may occur if the airway is compromised. C4 levels are typically low during an attack; they may be normal in between attacks.

Acquired angio-oedema is associated with allergic reactions, and is often associated with urticaria. Approximately 94% of cases of angio-oedema are drug-induced (most are patients taking ACE inhibitors). Insect stings and foods are other predisposing factors.

30 B: Henoch–Schönlein purpura

Henoch–Schönlein purpura (HSP) is characterised by the tissue deposition of IgA-containing immune complexes. The pathogenesis of this disorder may be similar to that of IgA nephropathy, which is associated with identical histologic findings in the kidney. HSP occurs more often in children than in adults, and many cases follow an upper respiratory tract infection, suggesting that the precipitating antigen may be infectious. The clinical manifestations include a classic tetrad that can occur in any order and at any time over a period of several days to several weeks: rash; arthralgias; abdominal pain; and renal disease. The rash is typically purpuric (with normal clotting studies) and distributed symmetrically over the lower legs and arms. Goodpasture's syndrome refers to the clinical constellation of glomerulonephritis, pulmonary haemorrhage, and anti-glomerular basement membrane (GBM) antibodies (IgG).

31 B: Hypomagnesaemia

Persistent hypocalcaemia and hyperphosphataemia, in the absence of renal failure or increased tissue breakdown, is virtually diagnostic of either hypoparathyroidism or pseudohypoparathyroidism. Hypomagnesaemia causes end-organ resistance to PTH and inhibits the hypocalcaemic feedback loop through uncertain mechanisms, leading to a state of functional hypoparathyroidism. Alcoholics become hypomagnesaemic partially by an osmotic diuresis from alcohol. Urinary losses have been reported to be two to three times control values. The albumin levels are normal and the calcium reading reflects the true calcium level and will match the corrected one. Hypoalbuminaemia might result in a false calcium reading which is lower than the corrected one. Poor dietary intake of calcium and intestinal malabsorption might lead to hypocalcaemia but the phosphate levels would also be low. Osteoporosis is not associated with bone profile abnormalities *per se*.

32 A: Action tremor

The presence of subtle bradykinesia (unblinking gaze and monotonous voice) or resting tremor in early cases of parkinsonism helps to make the diagnosis, although these signs may not appear until later on. Parkinson's disease is the most common cause of resting tremor. It is often described as 'pill-rolling' tremor. Action tremor is the main feature of essential tremor. Action tremor becomes immediately apparent when the arms are held outstretched and typically it increases at the very end of goal-directed movements, such as drinking from a glass.

33 A: Hereditary haemorrhagic telangiectasia

To make a definite diagnosis of HHT at least three of the following four criteria must present:

- Epistaxis, which is recurrent and spontaneous
- Multiple mucocutaneous telangiectases

- Visceral lesions, such as gastrointestinal or pulmonary arteriovenous malformations
- First-degree relative with HHT (diagnosed by these criteria).

The bleeding time is usually normal. Bleeding time is a measure of the interaction of platelets with the blood vessel wall. A prolonged bleeding time is seen in thrombocytopenia (platelet count usually below $50 \times 10^9/l$), in qualitative platelet abnormalities (as in uraemia and platelet storage-pool disease, and essential thrombocytosis), in von Willebrand's disease, in some cases of vascular purpura, and in severe fibrinogen deficiency, in which it is probably the result of platelet dysfunction.

34 D: Grand mal seizure

The blood picture is typical of megaloblastic anaemia. The recent onset of unsteady gait and sensory ataxia would suggest the diagnosis of vitamin B_{12} rather than folic acid deficiency. The neurological problems with B_{12} deficiency, when present, consist of the classic picture of subacute combined degeneration of the dorsal and lateral spinal columns. This lesion, specific for vitamin B_{12} deficiency, is due to a defect in myelin formation of unknown mechanism. The neuropathy is symmetrical and affects the legs more than the arms. It begins with paresthesiae and ataxia, associated with loss of vibration and position sense, and can progress to severe weakness, spasticity, clonus, paraplegia and even faecal and urinary incontinence. Other neurological abnormalities that may be seen are axonal degeneration of peripheral nerves and central nervous system symptoms, including memory loss, irritability and dementia. Patients may demonstrate Lhermitte's sign, a shock-like sensation that radiates to the feet during neck flexion. Not all patients with neurological abnormalities are anaemic or have a macrocytic picture. Seizures are not a feature associated with this disorder.

35 B: Pao$_2$ of 8 kPa

A history of hives, eczema, allergic rhinitis, blood and sputum eosinophilia, and nasal polyps may all suggest associated allergic diseases. These features are also associated with positive reversibility tests. Up to 30% of patients have an increase of 15% or more in their FEV_1 following inhalation of a β-agonist aerosol. However, the absence of a bronchodilator response during a single test never justifies withholding bronchodilator therapy. Hypoxia in itself is a constant feature of the disease and is not a reliable predictor of response to bronchodilators. Impaired oxygen diffusion capacity is a feature of emphysema where little or no reversibility is expected.

36   A: Muscle atrophy

Atrophy and fasciculations are common with lower motor neurone disease and unusual with upper motor neurone disease.

37   D: Syphilis

An Argyll Robertson pupil is caused by damage to cells in the pretectal region of the midbrain. As a result of this damage, signals carried by the optic nerve from the retina are not relayed via the pretectal nucleus on the affected side to the Edinger–Westphal nuclei. This results in a loss of both the direct and consensual pupillary light reflexes when light is shone into the eye on the affected side. Because the accommodation reflex pathway is distinct from the pupillary light reflex pathway the accommodation reflex is unaffected. The pupils are unequal and irregular.

Horner's syndrome results from sympathetic dysfunction of the eye, producing the classic combination of miosis, anhidrosis (depending on lesion location), and ptosis. Lesions anywhere along the sympathetic course (from the ipsilateral hypothalamus, through the brainstem and cervical cord, to the level of the C8–T1 roots, over the lung apex, up the carotid artery into the cavernous sinus, out of the superior orbital fissure, and through the orbit) may produce Horner's syndrome. Common causes include Wallenberg's lateral medullary syndrome (eg due to infarction), cervical cord disease (eg, syrinx, trauma), apical lung disease (eg Pancoast tumour). The pupil in third nerve palsy appears larger and poorly reactive to light and accommodation. Causes of oculomotor palsy include life-threatening conditions such as uncal herniation and aneurysmal compression (eg posterior communicating artery syndrome).

The Holmes–Adie pupil is a tonic pupil. Classically, the affected pupil is larger than the other and it is poorly reactive to light. The pupil reacts vigorously to accommodation, constituting one of the accommodation–light dissociation syndromes. The pupil's better response to accommodation than to a light stimulus occurs because the lesion involves the more dorsally located fibres that serve the pupillary response to light and spares the more ventrally located fibres that serve the pupillary response to accommodation. Usually it is a unilateral phenomenon without pathological significance. It is most common in women aged 20–40 years. It is commonly associated with a loss of knee jerks. Extraocular movements are normal and there is no ptosis.

38 D: Wilson's disease
Wilson's disease (hepatolenticular degeneration) is an autosomal recessive defect in cellular copper transport. Neurological disorders are present in up to 35% of patients with Wilson's disease. Signs include a parkinsonian-like tremor, rigidity, clumsiness of gait, slurring of speech, inappropriate and uncontrollable grinning (risus sardonicus) and drooling. Asymptomatic hepatic involvement is usually present. Patients with Wilson's disease most often present with liver disease (which can range from asymptomatic elevations in the serum aminotransferase or bilirubin concentrations to fulminant hepatic failure, to chronic hepatitis. Patients in whom Wilson's disease is suspected should have a slit-lamp examination for detection of Kayser–Fleischer rings. Wilson's disease should be suspected when unexplained liver or neuropsychiatric disease are encountered in a young person under the age of 30.

Parkinson's disease typically presents in middle and late life. However, early-onset disease can occur before the age of 40, and a juvenile form presents before the age of 20. Most affected children have a rigid, akinetic disorder, although many have a typical resting tremor. Huntington's disease typically presents during the fourth and fifth decades of life. However, onset occurs during childhood or adolescence in approximately 10% of affected patients. Huntington's disease is transmitted as an autosomal dominant trait. Patients with juvenile-onset Huntington's disease develop dystonia, ataxia, and seizures. Neither Parkinson's disease nor Huntington's disease are associated with liver or eye disorders.

39 D: Seborrhoeic dermatitis
Seborrhoeic dermatitis is characterised by erythema and mild epidermal hyperproliferation leading to scaliness. The scalp and face are most commonly affected. Seborrhoeic dermatitis is a common presenting feature in patients with HIV infection. Up to 40% of HIV-seropositive individuals and 80% of those with AIDS suffer from this skin disorder. Clinicians should consider HIV infection in any patient presenting with a new onset of severe seborrhoeic dermatitis.

40 B: Splenomegaly occurs in 20% of cases
Haemorrhage is the most common cause of excessive loss of body iron, but it can occur with haemoglobinuria from intravascular haemolysis. The bone marrow is stimulated to increase production of haemoglobin, thereby depleting iron in body stores. Once stores are depleted, haemoglobin synthesis is impaired and microcytic

hypochromic erythrocytes are produced. Often, the platelet count is elevated (>450 × 10⁹/l). This normalises following iron therapy. Low serum iron and ferritin levels with an elevated total iron-binding capacity (TIBC) are diagnostic of iron deficiency. While a low serum ferritin is virtually diagnostic of iron deficiency, a normal serum ferritin may be seen in patients who are deficient in iron and have coexistent disease (hepatitis, anaemia of chronic disorders). A bone marrow aspirate can be diagnostic of iron deficiency. The absence of stainable iron in a bone marrow aspirate is an early feature and permits establishment of a diagnosis of iron deficiency without other laboratory tests. Splenomegaly occurs in 15–25% of cases.

41 D: Cavernous sinus thrombosis

The picture is one of severe infection around the left eye associated with increased retro-orbital pressure, probably resulting from venous congestion. The loss of sensation in the forehead and ophthalmoplegia indicate lesions of the ophthalmic (V1) branch of the trigeminal nerve and the oculomotor nerve (third cranial nerve) or trochlear or fourth cranial nerve. This clinical picture is typical of cavernous sinus thrombosis.

A number of cranial nerves are located in fibrous sheaths along the lateral wall of each cavernous sinus: the ophthalmic (V1) and maxillary (V2) branches of the trigeminal nerve. The abducent nerve is located more medially, near the internal carotid artery, which also tracks through the cavernous sinus.

Approximately 50% of cases of septic cavernous sinus thrombosis are preceded by facial infections. Nasal furuncles are the most common facial infection to produce this complication, particularly if the furuncle is squeezed or drained in the absence of antibiotic coverage. Headache is the most common early symptom and generally precedes fever and periorbital oedema by several days. The symptoms of cavernous sinus thrombosis are not specific, but the presence of cranial nerve signs on physical examination in a patient with headache should alert the clinician to the possibility of the diagnosis.

Given the large size of the superior sagittal sinus, septic thrombotic occlusion is very rare. Occlusion of the anterior segment in association with frontal sinusitis presents with mild to moderate headache and spontaneously resolves following the development of collateral venous channels. The most common infection associated with complete occlusion of the superior sagittal sinus is bacterial meningitis. Septic thrombosis of the superior sagittal sinus results in haemorrhagic infarcts, due to cortical vein thrombosis, and communicating hydrocephalus. When combined with the cerebral oedema associated with meningitis, massive brain infarction and death commonly ensue.

Periorbital cellulitis and osteomyelitis of the left maxillary sinus might produce chemosis, swelling and cyanosis of the upper face but is rarely associated with cranial nerve injury. Left retro-orbital tumour would cause headache, proptosis and diplopia from pressure and displacement of the eyeball but it is not associated with signs of infection or any specific cranial nerve involvement.

42 A: Factor XIII deficiency

Factor XIII deficiency leads to the prevention of forming a stable fibrin clot. The clinical hallmark of this disorder is delayed bleeding after surgery or an invasive procedure, because the initial clot is mechanically weak. Large spontaneous haematomas or intracranial haemorrhage can occur. Most patients are over the age 50 and death from bleeding is not uncommon. Factor XIII deficiency produces a unique pattern on coagulation testing. The PT and APTT are normal, but the urea clot solubilty assay is abnormal, because the absence of fibrin crosslinking causes the clot to lyse much more rapidly in 5 M urea. All the other bleeding disorders listed are associated with abnormal coagulation tests. Protein C deficiency is not associated with bleeding tendency.

43 E: Chickenpox might rapidly progress to severe and fatal haemorrhagic varicella

Neutropenia is defined as an absolute neutrophil count (ANC) of less than $1.5 \times 10^9/l$. The drugs with the highest risk of inducing severe neutropenia include carbizamole and propylthiouracil. It appears to cause neutropenia by immune-mediated destruction of circulating neutrophils. Neutropenia may present days to weeks after beginning the drug and is often acute with explosive symptoms. Rechallenge, or inadvertent subsequent administration, is associated with a prompt recurrence with even small doses. Recurrent infections are the only significant consequence of neutropenia. However, the classic signs of infection are often less evident in patients with neutropenia. Endogenous bacterial flora are the most common pathogens, including *Staphylococcus aureus* from the skin and Gram-negative organisms from the gastrointestinal and urinary tracts. Common sites of infection include the oral cavity and mucous membranes, the skin, and perianal and genital areas. With persistent severe neutropenia systemic infection occurs, associated with bacteraemia. The risk of severe or fatal chickenpox disease increases in adults and in patients with depressed T-cell immunity (eg lymphoreticular malignancy) or in those receiving corticosteroids or chemotherapy. Isolated neutropenia does not increase the susceptibility to viral or parasitic infection.

44 A: Osteoporotic vertebral collapse fracture may be responsible for his backache
Multiple myeloma is the most common primary neoplasm of the skeletal system. The disease is a malignancy of plasma cells. Radiologically, multiple destructive lesions of the skeleton as well as severe demineralisation characterise multiple myeloma. Since bone loss occurs mostly in the axial skeleton, patients with myeloma are at risk for compression fractures of the spine and pathological fractures of the major weight-bearing bones of the body. The classic presentation is low back pain in an older man, with subsequent discovery of demineralisation or a myelomatous deposit.

45 B: Bullous pemphigoid
Bullous pemphigoid is a chronic, blistering autoimmune disease of unknown cause that most commonly affects the over 60s. Tense bullae commonly occur in the flexural areas, groin, and axillae. Oral involvement occurs in one-third of cases but is rarely the presenting feature. Pemphigus vulgaris is characterised by flaccid bullae that typically begin in the oropharynx and may then spread to involve the skin. In pemphigus vulgaris, mucous membrane involvement is more common and intact bullae are rare. Skin biopsy for routine and direct immunofluorescence is needed to confirm the diagnosis. Dermatitis herpetiformis is characterised by grouped vesicles with extensor rather than flexural distribution. Herpes zoster rash initially appears along the dermatome as grouped vesicles or bullae which evolve into pustular or occasionally haemorrhagic lesions within three to four days. The hallmark of Stevens–Johnson syndrome is the development of large blisters in the mouth, in the throat, on the skin, around the anus or genitals, or even on the eyes.

46 C: Absence of excessive bleeding after tooth extraction
Haemophilia A and B are X-linked recessive diseases. They exhibit a range of clinical severity that correlates well with assayed factor levels. Severe disease is defined as <1% factor activity, whereas 1–5% and >5% of normal are defined as moderate and mild disease, respectively. A normal platelet count, normal PT and a prolonged APTT are characteristic of haemophilia A and haemophilia B. However, patients with mild haemophilia B may have normal or near normal APTTs. Thus, in undiagnosed mild

bleeding disorders, a factor IX assay should be performed even if the APTT is normal.

Approximately one-third of patients with haemophilia have a negative family history. As many as one-third of patients with mild disease (factor levels 5%) have very few or no bleeding episodes, which, as noted above, occur only with trauma or surgery. They seldom bleed from small cuts or venepuncture but delayed bleeding can occur in patients with mild haemophilia after minor surgical procedures such as tooth extraction. Patients who undergo similar procedures without a haemorrhage or delayed bleeding are very unlikely to be suffering from haemophilia.

47 E: Contact isolation

MRSA infection usually develops in hospitalised patients who are elderly or very sick or who have an open wound (such as a bedsore) or a tube going into their body (such as a urinary catheter or intravenous catheter). MRSA causes illness in people outside hospitals and healthcare facilities as well. Cases of MRSA disease in the community have been associated with recent antibiotic use, sharing contaminated items, having active skin diseases, and living in crowded settings. Staphylococcal bacteria and MRSA can spread among people having close contact with infected people. MRSA is almost always spread by direct physical contact, and not through the air. Spread may also occur through indirect contact by touching objects (ie, towels, sheets, wound dressings, clothes, workout areas, sports equipment) contaminated by the infected skin of a person with MRSA or staphylococcal bacteria.

Use standard precautions plus:

- Place the patient in a private room or with someone with the same infection if possible.
- Use gloves when entering the room. Change gloves after contact with infective material.
- Use a gown when entering the room if contact with the patient is anticipated or if the patient has diarrhoea, a colostomy or wound drainage not covered by a dressing.
- Limit the movement or transport of the patient from the room.
- Ensure that patient-care items, bedside equipment, and frequently touched surfaces receive daily cleaning.
- Dedicate use of non-critical patient-care equipment to a single patient, or cohort of patients with the same pathogen. If this is not feasible, adequate disinfection between patients is necessary.

48 D: Behçet's disease

Behçet's disease is a chronic, multisystem autoimmune disease that involves inflammation of blood vessels throughout the body, characterised by the triad of aphthous stomatitis, genital ulcers, and uveitis. Genital ulcers can be found on the scrotum, penile shaft or glans. In women, they are found on the labium minor, the cervix, or vaginal wall. Ulcers may be painless in the last two sites. These are not herpes, therefore they do not blister and they are virus negative. Behçet's disease is not infectious, contagious, or sexually transmitted. Phlebitis or arteritis occurs in as many as a quarter of the patients and predisposes to thrombosis or aneurysms.

Granuloma inguinale, a sexually transmitted chronic infection of the skin and subcutaneous tissue of the genitalia, perineum, and inguinal area, has an incubation period of 2–3 months. The infective agent is *Calymmatobacterium granulomatis*. A painful papule is the first sign of granuloma inguinale which develops into large, usually painless, spreading, exuberant ulcers. In primary syphilis genital ulcer chancre is usually single with nodular base.

49 E: Intravenous adrenaline (epinephrine)

The treatment of acute inhalation-related injury and illness is generally supportive. Acute dysrhythmias should be treated according to established protocols. The use of sympathomimetics, such as adrenaline (epinephrine), noradrenaline (norepinephrine), or isoprenaline should be avoided in patients with ventricular fibrillation. β-blockers should be administered early to protect the catecholamine-sensitised heart.

50 D: More than 50% of patients stayed four days or more

The large SD (relative to the mean) and the fact that the median is much smaller than the mean indicate that length of stay does not follow a Normal distribution and in fact is positively skewed.

A is incorrect because the mean does not (for a non-Normal distribution) split the data-set into two halves; the median does

B is incorrect because the data follow a positively skewed distribution

C is highly likely to be incorrect because the range cannot be determined from the information supplied in the question (it is not defined by $2 \times SD$)

D is correct because the median is given as 5 days. Hence at least 50% of patients stayed 5 days or longer, thus more than 50% stayed 4 days or longer

E is incorrect because, as the data are non-Normal, the usual formula, '95% of patients have length of stay with $+/- 2 \times SD$ of the mean', does not apply.

51 D: Hebephrenic schizophrenia

The EEG can be a useful investigation in apparent psychosis or behavioural disturbance. EEGs in interictal psychosis are abnormal in the majority of cases. Herpes simplex encephalitis and subacute panencephalitis are associated with periodic complexes. Metabolic encephalopathy is associated with frontal intermittent rhythmic delta activity. Subtypes of schizophrenia are not commonly associated with EEG abnormalities.

52 B: Pyoderma gangrenosum

Pyoderma gangrenosum is an ulcerating skin disease, which generally presents with chronic non-healing necrotising ulcers, most frequently on the lower extremities. The typical onset is with a tender, erythematous macule, papule or pustule, which subsequently ulcerates. Not infrequently the lesions arise in areas of trauma. Pyoderma gangrenosum may also be associated with several systemic diseases, most notably inflammatory bowel disease, as well as rheumatoid arthritis, chronic active hepatitis and IgA monoclonal gammopathy. The classic clinical appearance is of a necrotic ulcer with a purulent base and a violaceous, undermined border. The lesions will persist for months to years and if not properly diagnosed and treated may lead to unnecessary and ineffective skin grafts and amputations. There are no specific laboratory abnormalities associated with the condition and no definitive histopathological findings. Treatment consists of systemic corticosteroids for advanced lesions. Early lesions may benefit from the use of intralesional steroids as well.

53 A: Alcoholic cardiomyopathy

Measurement of the jugular venous pressure may be an important distinguishing feature in determining whether ascites is due to alcoholic cardiomyopathy or cirrhosis. The jugular venous pressure is typically normal or low-normal in cirrhosis. A low or normal jugular venous pressure therefore makes heart failure much less likely as the cause of ascites. On the other hand, in the absence of tense ascites, an elevated jugular venous pressure is highly suggestive of a contribution from cardiac dysfunction.

54 A: Splenomegaly

Schistosomiasis may be one of the most common causes of portal hypertension worldwide. The two major species producing liver infection are *Schistosoma mansoni* and *Schistosoma japonicum*. Chronic schistosomiasis can present with predominantly intestinal or hepatointestinal manifestations. The liver disease is characterised by portal hypertension, hepatomegaly, and often marked splenomegaly, which can lead to variceal haemorrhage and hypersplenism. The number and distribution of the varices are similar to other causes of portal hypertension. In children, chronic infection is associated with growth retardation. Ascites is relatively uncommon and, when it occurs, is usually mild. Liver function is invariably preserved, and liver failure or hepatic encephalopathy almost never occurs.

55 C: HIV infection
The immune response of the host is an important determinant of the type of infection caused by *Candida*. Cellular immune deficiency states including, HIV/acquired immunodeficiency syndrome (AIDS) are important predisposing factors for *Candida* infection. AIDS should be suspected in an otherwise healthy individual who presents with oropharyngeal candidiasis. Antibiotic use, chemotherapy or radiation therapy are other predisposing factors. Oropharyngeal candidiasis is often associated with more advanced stages of lymphomas.

56 E: Give intravenous atropine sulphate (0.6 mg)
Sinus bradycardia can be defined as a sinus rhythm with a resting heart rate of 60 bpm or less. However, few patients actually become symptomatic until their heart rate drops to less than 50 bpm. In symptomatic patients, intravenous atropine may be used.

57 C: Liver abscess
The organism of the *Streptococcus milleri* group are commensals, commonly isolated from the mouth, oropharynx, gastrointestinal tract and vagina, and responsible for a variety of human and animal infections. *S. milleri* is regularly found with anaerobes in abscesses in the brain, liver, lung and gut.

58 C: Vancomycin
The level of renal function below which the dose of a drug must be reduced depends on whether the drug is eliminated entirely by renal excretion or is partly metabolised, and how toxic it is. The dosing interval is determined by the creatinine clearance. When the creatinine clearance is below 30 ml/min (normal range 75–125 ml/min) the dosing interval is 72 hours for vancomycin and 24 hours for gentamicin. Penicillins and cephalosporins are associated with minor dose-related side effects and therefore limited alteration in dosing interval might prove to be necessary in certain situations.

59 E: Right heart failure

Patients with right-sided heart failure have peripheral oedema and, in severe cases, anasarca with ascites and oedema of the abdominal wall. Shortness of breath is commonly present and may be due to underlying pulmonary disease or coexistent left ventricular failure. The oedema in these disorders is due to an increase in venous pressure behind the right side of the heart. Thus, the pressures in the right atrium and subclavian vein are elevated, changes that can be detected by estimation of the jugular venous pressure or by direct measurement with a central venous pressure catheter. The hepatojugular reflux is often positive in these circumstances.

60 D: Sphenoid wing meningioma

Foster Kennedy syndrome is characterised by papilloedema in one eye and optic atrophy in the other. It results from the simultaneous presence of raised intracranial pressure and optic nerve compression secondary to tumour – classically due to a meningioma of the olfactory groove or more commonly, due to a meningioma of the sphenoid wing. Papilloedema in both eyes is a characteristic feature of raised intracranial pressure caused by the other options given, where compression of the optic nerve is not a feature.

61 D: Barrett's oesophagus

The majority of oesophageal cancers are squamous cell carcinoma or adenocarcinoma. Barrett's oesophagus is a condition in which abnormal columnar epithelium replaces the stratified squamous epithelium that normally lines the distal oesophagus. It is the most severe histological consequence of chronic gastro-oesophageal reflux disease (GORD) and predisposes to the development of adenocarcinoma of the oesophagus. Most oesophageal adenocarcinomas arise from Barrett's metaplasia.

62 E: Hypocalcaemia

Rhabdomyolysis is a common disorder which may result from a large variety of diseases, trauma, or toxic insults to skeletal muscle. It may be defined as a clinical and biochemical syndrome resulting from an injury which damages the integrity of the sarcolemma of skeletal muscle, leading to the release of potentially toxic muscle cell components into the circulation This may result in potentially life-threatening complications, including myoglobinuric acute renal failure, hyperkalaemia, cardiac arrest, disseminated intravascular coagulation and, more locally, compartment syndrome. The primary diagnostic indicator of rhabdomyolysis is an elevated serum creatine phosphokinase (CK) to at least five times the normal value. This elevation is generally to such a degree that myocardial infarction and other causes of a raised CK are excluded. Additionally, the CK-MM isoenzyme predominates in rhabdomyolysis, comprising at least 98% of the total value. The other important finding frequently seen in rhabdomyolysis is myoglobinuria which produces visible pigmenturia (classically a cola-coloured urine). It may be caused by toxins (alcohol, statins, barbiturates, amphetamines, heroin, phenmetrazine, methadone or metabolic disorders (diabetic ketoacidosis, non-ketotic hyperosmolar coma, hypothyroidism, hypophosphatemia, hyponatraemia, hypokalaemia.

63 B: Allergic bronchopulmonary aspergillosis

Allergic bronchopulmonary aspergillosis (ABPA) is a complex hypersensitivity reaction in patients with asthma which occurs when bronchi become colonised by *Aspergillus*. Repeated episodes of bronchial obstruction, inflammation, and mucoid impaction can lead to bronchiectasis. The chest X-ray may show parenchymal infiltrates and/or bronchiectasis (usually involving the upper lobes for unknown reasons). Peripheral blood eosinophilia $> 0.5 \times 10^9/l$ is often present. Although other causes of pulmonary eosinophilia are characterised by blood eosinophilia and chest infiltrate they rarely progress to bronchiectasis.

64 D: Anaerobic bacteria

In lung abscesses, anaerobes are recovered in up to 90% of the patients, 50% of patients show a mixture of anaerobes and aerobes. The most common anaerobes are *Peptostreptococcus*, *Bacteroides*, *Fusobacterium* species, and microaerophilic streptococci. Lung abscesses are usually caused by aspiration of infected material from the upper airway. Other organisms that may infrequently cause lung abscess include *Staphylococcus aureus*, *Streptococcus pyogenes*, *Streptococcus pneumoniae* (rarely), *Klebsiella pneumoniae*, *Haemophilus influenzae*, *Actinomyces* species, *Nocardia* species, and Gram-negative bacilli.

65 E: Gentamicin

Pseudomembranous colitis is due to infection by *Clostridium difficile*, a Gram-positive anaerobic bacillus. Ten per cent of patients on antibiotics develop diarrhoea; only 1% develop pseudomembranous colitis. Those with mild diarrhoea should have their antibiotics stopped. If colitis is present they need active treatment with oral antibiotics: metronidazole (first-line therapy) and vancomycin (second-line therapy). Symptoms usually improve within 72 hours but it may take 10 days for the diarrhoea to stop. Oral treatment with antimicrobial agents effective against *C. difficile* is the preferred treatment. No reliable parenteral treatment for pseudomembranous colitis exists. As alternative therapy, bacitracin, teicoplanin and colestyramine are also considered in individual cases.

66 A: Mitral stenosis and tricuspid regurgitation

A loud first heart sound and a diastolic rumble are the main features of isolated mitral stenosis. In more advanced cases secondary pulmonary hypertension will ensue. The right ventricle will soon dilate and its function will become compromised. With time this will lead to tricuspid regurgitation identified clinically by a large v wave in the jugular pulse.

67 C: Multiple sclerosis (MS)

Plaques suggestive of MS are typically found on MRI in the periventricular region, corpus callosum, centrum semiovale and, to a lesser extent, in the deep white matter structures and basal ganglia. In Friedreich's ataxia the MRI typically reveals spinal cord (and, in some cases, cerebellar) atrophy. The variety of neurological manifestations in patients with syphilis is wide, a feature that helps explain why this infection is known as 'the great imitator'. In meningovascular syphilis the clinical manifestations depend upon which vessel is occluded. Aphasia and/or hemiparesis are most common. In tabes dorsalis typical manifestations include paresthesiae, abnormal gait and lightning (sudden and severe) pains of the extremities or trunk. It is a disease of the posterior columns of the spinal cord and of the dorsal roots. The MRI features in Huntington's disease generally include generalised brain atrophy.

68 D: Anti-smooth muscle antibodies

The clinical picture is typical of chronic hepatitis. The patient's age and the other manifestations, such as fatiguability, lethargy, malaise and especially arthralgia involving the small joints, are characteristic clinical features of autoimmune hepatitis (AIH). Anti-smooth muscle antibodies are directed against actin and non-actin components, including tubulin, vimentin, desmin, and skeletin and are standard markers of AIH. They are present in 87% of patients with AIH.

Antimitochondrial antibodies are the serological hallmark of primary biliary cirrhosis. Caeruloplasmin levels are typically low in patients with Wilson's disease. Anti-parietal cell antibodies are associated with many autoimmune disorders, including pernicious anaemia and hypothyroidism. They are not specific, and may even be less sensitive: as a result, their usefulness in diagnosing pernicious anaemia has been called into question. Viral hepatitis is a possible diagnosis, however the presence of musculoskelatal symptoms at the outset of the disease and the fact that this patient was suffering from hypothyroidism indicates an organ-specific autoimmune process rather than a viral infection.

69 B: 24-hour pH monitoring of the lower oesophagus

The most common causes of chronic cough are postnasal drip, asthma and gastro-oesophageal reflux. Many patients complain of symptoms of gastro-oesophageal reflux (heartburn or a sour taste in the mouth) but these symptoms are absent In more than 40% of patients in whom cough is due to reflux. The possible mechanisms include: stimulation of receptors in the upper respiratory tract (eg in the larynx); aspiration of gastric contents; or an oesophageal tracheobronchial cough reflex induced by reflux of acid into the distal oesophagus. The presence of cough induced by gastro-oesophageal reflux may be suggested by an abnormal barium swallow, but this study is negative in the majority of patients. Prolonged (24-hour) oesophageal pH monitoring, ideally performed with event markers to allow correlation of cough with oesophageal pH, is generally considered the best optimal diagnostic study, with a sensitivity exceeding 90%.

70 C: Steatorrhoea is likely to develop as a result of pancreatic insufficiency

This patient has inflammatory bowel disease or IBD (ulcerative colitis or Crohn's disease). A major concern in the evolution of ulcerative colitis is the potential for the development of colon cancer. The risk of acquiring colon cancer is related to both the duration and extent of the disease. The incidence of colon cancer begins to increase relative to the general population some seven to eight years after the onset of disease in those patients with disease which extends beyond the splenic flexure.

Gallstones are seen in 13–34% of patients with ileitis or ileal resection. They are probably caused by the malabsorption of bile acids, which interferes with their enterohepatic circulation. This leads to depletion of bile salts and the formation of lithogenic bile. First-degree relatives of patients with IBD are approximately three to twenty times more likely to develop the disease than the general population. However, the substantial majority of patients (>85%) have no family history of IBD.

Fat malabsorption may be seen in 30–40% of patients with Crohn's disease. The cause is multifactorial, including small bowel inflammation, decreased bowel length due to surgery, bacterial overgrowth, bile acid deficiency due to disease or resection of the terminal ileum, or the use of medicines such as colestyramine that bind bile acids. Pancreatic function is usually maintained.

71 B: Alcoholic hepatitis

Alcoholic hepatitis is a syndrome of progressive inflammatory liver injury associated with chronic heavy intake of ethanol. Patients who are affected severely present with subacute onset of fever, hepatomegaly, leukocytosis, and marked impairment of liver function (eg jaundice, coagulopathy). Alcoholic hepatitis usually persists and progresses to cirrhosis if heavy alcohol use continues. Liver enzymes exhibit a characteristic pattern. In most patients, the AST is elevated moderately, while the ALT is normal or only mildly elevated. This is the opposite of what is observed in most other liver diseases. An AST/ALT ratio greater than 1 is almost universal in alcoholic hepatitis. Even in severe disease, the elevations of aminotransferases are modest, and an AST greater than 500 U/l should raise the suspicion of an alternative diagnosis. An AST/ALT ratio greater than 1 may accompany cirrhosis of any cause and therefore is less diagnostically specific in the setting of cirrhosis.

72 D: Polymyalgia rheumatica

A variety of medical and surgical conditions can result in reactive thrombocytosis. These include iron deficiency anaemia, surgical or functional asplenia, metastatic cancer, trauma (surgical or otherwise), acute bleeding or haemolysis, and a variety of infectious and inflammatory processes. When a cause for reactive thrombocytosis is not readily apparent, the demonstration of elevated acute phase reactants (C-reactive protein or CRP, fibrinogen, erythrocyte sedimentation rate) may be used as evidence for the presence of an occult inflammatory process.

73 E: Paroxysmal nocturnal haemoglobinuria

This blood picture is typical of haemolytic anaemia.There are many causes of haemolytic anaemia, but there are, broadly, two categories: acquired and inherited. In general iron stores are not depleted in haemolytic anaemias and iron supplementation should not be given. The exception is when there is intravascular haemolysis and the haemoglobin is lost from the circulation outside the body (in the urine) as in paroxysmal nocturnal haemoglobinuria.

74 A: Dapsone

Methaemoglobin is an altered state of haemoglobin in which the ferrous (Fe^{2+}) irons of haem are oxidised to the ferric (Fe^{3+}) state. The ferric haem of methaemoglobin is unable to bind oxygen. Methaemoglobinaemia may be clinically suspected by the presence of clinical cyanosis in the face of a normal arterial PO_2 (PaO_2). Methaemoglobinaemia may be congenital or acquired. The acquired form is often caused by drugs, such as dapsone, nitrates, aniline dyes, chloroquine or primaquine.

75 C: von Willebrand's disease

This patient has an inherited bleeding disorder. A positive history in a female member of the family is an exclusive sign of autosomal inherited disorders. Haemophilia A and haemophilia B are inherited as sex-linked diseases. Idiopathic thrombocytopenic purpura is not inherited and lupus anticoagulant is not associated with an increased bleeding tendency. von Willebrand's disease is the most common inherited bleeding disorder, affecting up to 1% of the population. von Willebrand named the disorder hereditary pseudohaemophilia because he recognised the autosomal inheritance pattern in family members (in contrast to the sex-linked recessive pattern seen in the haemophilias).

76 A: Haemarthrosis

Haemophilia A and haemophilia B are X-linked recessive diseases. They exhibit a range of clinical severity that correlates well with assayed factor levels. Severe disease is defined as <1% factor activity, whereas 1–5% and >5% of normal are defined as moderate and mild disease respectively. The hallmark of haemophilia is haemorrhage into the joints. Haemarthrosis is the most common presentation in severe adult haemophilia. Severe haemophilia (defined as less than 1% of normal factor activity) causes haemarthrosis in 75–90% of patients. The knee is the most common joint involved, followed by the elbow, ankle, hip, and shoulder. Bilateral involvement is not uncommon.

77 D: α_1 Antitrypsin deficiency

The main clinical manifestations of α_1-antitrypsin (AAT) deficiency relate to three separate organs: the lung, the liver and, much less often, the skin. In the lung, severe deficiency of AAT predisposes to chronic obstructive pulmonary disease, especially pan-acinar emphysema. Liver disorders, such as neonatal hepatitis, cirrhosis both in children and adults, and hepatocellular carcinoma are associated with some AAT-deficient phenotypes. Approximately 10–15% of adults develop chronic hepatic disease.

78 D: Sickle cell disease
The spleen is usually small and non-functioning in most adult cases of sickle cell disease. Fibrosis of the spleen results from repeated vaso-occlusive ischaemic episodes over the years.

79 D: Pityriasis rosea
Pityriasis rosea is a self-limiting, inflammatory dermatosis of unknown cause. It characteristically presents with oval, scaly, tannish-pink patches or plaques on the trunk, the generalised eruption being preceded by a single lesion (called a 'herald patch') by days to weeks. Typically, the lesions follow the skin cleavage lines in a pattern that has been likened to that of a Christmas tree. The lesions usually disappear within two months without any treatment.

80 B: Liver cirrhosis
Patients with liver disease often show spur cells (the extreme form of acanthocytes), echinocytes (also called 'burr cells') and target cells on the peripheral blood smear. These changes are most severe in advanced hepatocellular disease, which may be associated with 20–30% acanthocytes in the peripheral blood and moderate to severe haemolysis.

81 C: Thrombotic thrombocytopenic purpura (TTP)
The syndrome of thrombotic thrombocytopenic purpura (TTP) is characterised by thrombocytopenia, microangiopathic haemolytic anaemia and renal disease. Neurological manifestations and fever complete the pentad of symptoms characteristic of TTP. The diagnosis requires the presence of at least two major criteria (ie thrombocytopenia, microangiopathic anaemia or neurological dysfunction) and two minor criteria (ie fever, renal dysfunction or circulating thrombi). Profound thrombocytopenia develops because platelets clump in the microcirculation faster than they are produced by megakaryocytes in the bone marrow. Platelet counts commonly drop below $20 \times 10^9/l$, and often below $10 \times 10^9/l$.

The platelet clumps reversibly occlude microcirculatory vessels, causing transient ischaemia of organ systems. Ischaemic symptoms may involve any organ, but CNS involvement is especially common. The presentation may include anything from memory disturbance, behavioural irregularities or headaches, to coma. Raised serum LDH is the hallmark of intravascular red cell destruction in TTP. LDH levels also rise as tissues in ischaemic areas become necrotic and so the increased LDH also may derive from dying myocardial, cerebral, pulmonary, renal, or other cells.

Idiopathic thrombocytopenia (ITP) and aplastic anaemia are associated with thrombocytopenia and anaemia but not with intravascular haemolysis. Thalassaemia major and autoimmune haemolytic anaemia are not associated with thrombocytopenia and the haemolysis in both disorders is extravascular and therefore not associated with schistocytes in the peripheral blood.

82 A: Acid haemolysis test

The clinical syndrome of paroxysmal nocturnal haemoglobinuria (PNH) can present with three types of symptoms: with an acquired intracorpuscular haemolytic anaemia due to the abnormal susceptibility of the red cell membrane to the haemolytic activity of complement; with thromboses in large vessels (eg hepatic, abdominal, cerebral, and subdermal veins); or with a deficiency in haematopoiesis that may be mild or severe, as in pancytopenia in aplastic anaemia. The triad of haemolytic anaemia, pancytopenia and thrombosis makes PNH a unique clinical syndrome.

PNH is currently reclassified from being purely an acquired haemolytic anaemia due to a haematopoietic stem cell mutation defect to a haemolytic anaemia due to intravascular destruction of red blood cells (RBCs) by complement to varying degrees. The tests involved in establishing the diagnosis demonstrate the presence of RBCs that are exceptionally sensitive to the haemolytic action of complement. Acidified serum lysis and Ham's test are reliable ways to diagnose PNH.

83 D: Hypercalcaemia

Constipation is the most common gastrointestinal complaint in patients with hypercalcaemia of any cause. Anorexia and vague abdominal complaints are also common symptoms. Chronic hypercalcaemia leads to a defect in renal concentrating ability that may induce polyuria and polydipsia. Morphine causes lethargy, vomiting and constipation but does not lead to polyuria or polydipsia.

84 A: All the sons will be normal

Haemophilia is an X-linked recessive disease so all sons born to an affected father and normal mother will be normal, and all daughters born to an affected father and a normal mother will be carriers.

85 A: Alzheimer's disease

Dementia affects approximately 5% of people over 65 and 20% of individuals over 80 years. Alzheimer's disease accounts for around 60% of all cases of dementia, and usually has an insidious onset with gradual progression, without vascular risk factors. Depression is an important differential diagnosis in an older person presenting with memory impairment and apathy. Lewy body dementia accounts for approximately 20% of cases of dementia, and usually presents with Parkinsonism, fluctuating cognitive impairment and visual hallucinations. Mild cognitive impairment (MCI) is impairment of memory with preservation of other domains of cognition and intact activities of daily living. 30% of people with MCI will develop dementia within two years.

86 D: Diffusing capacity for carbon monoxide (D_{LCO})

Physiological pulmonary changes in morbid obesity reflect the impaired chest wall and lung compliance and the FVC, FEV_1, ERV, FRC, maximum voluntary ventilation and forced expiratory flow during the mid-expiratory phase are all significantly reduced. However, no abnormality in D_{LCO} is expected.

87 D: Tetany

Alkalosis enhances and acidosis depresses renal potassium secretion, probably by inducing corresponding changes in tubular cell potassium. Chloride is required for bicarbonate secretion in the collecting duct via a bicarbonate–chloride exchanger. In acute metabolic acidosis, hyperventilation is usual and may be intense (Kussmaul respiration), leading to washout of CO_2 and reduction in Pa_{CO_2}.

88 C: DNA

Ionising radiation produces biological effects by imparting energy to tissues and causing DNA damage with consequent loss of cellular reproductive ability.

89 C: β-Thalassaemia

Approximately 2.5% of the haemoglobin in normal red cells is Hb $\alpha_2\delta_2$. It can be readily separated from Hb A by electrophoresis or ion-exchange chromatography. The percentage of Hb A_2 is increased in β-thalassaemia, a finding that is a useful diagnostic aid. Hb A_2 is also slightly increased in megaloblastic anaemia. Hb A_2 is decreased in α-thalassaemia, iron deficiency and sideroblastic anaemias. In β-thalassemia major there is a complete failure of β-chain production. Hence there is very little, if any, Hb A present.

δ- and γ-chain production is increased. As a result there are raised levels of Hb A$_2$ and Hb F. Sickle cell homozygotes produce mainly haemoglobin S with variable amounts of fetal haemoglobin and haemoglobin A$_2$. Hereditary spherocytosis does not alter Hb A$_2$ production.

90   C: Kaposi's sarcoma

Epstein–Barr virus (EBV) is a widely disseminated herpesvirus which is spread by intimate contact between susceptible people and asymptomatic EBV shedders. The majority of primary EBV infections throughout the world are subclinical. Antibodies to EBV have been demonstrated in all population groups with a worldwide distribution: approximately 90–95% of adults are EBV-seropositive. EBV is the primary agent of infectious mononucleosis. It has been causally linked to a variety of malignancies and to lymphomas in transplant recipients. These include Burkitt's lymphoma, tumours in HIV-infected patients, Hodgkin's disease, nasopharyngeal and other head and neck carcinomas, and T cell lymphoma. Other EBV-induced diseases in HIV-positive individuals include oral hairy leukoplakia (OHL). The OHL lesions appear to be relatively specific for HIV and they are rarely seen in patients with other immunodeficiencies. Kaposi's sarcoma is a low-grade vascular tumour associated with human herpesvirus 8 (HHV-8).

91   B: Cholesterol

Bilirubin is formed by breakdown of haem present in haemoglobin, myoglobin, cytochromes, catalase, peroxidase and tryptophan pyrrolase. 80% of the daily bilirubin production (250–400 mg in adults) is derived from haemoglobin, the remaining 20% being contributed by other haemoproteins and rapid turnover of a small pool of free haem. Enhanced bilirubin formation is found in all conditions associated with increased red cell turnover such as intramedullary or intravascular haemolysis (eg haemolytic, dyserythropoietic and megaloblastic anaemias). Cholesterol does not contain haem in its structure.

92   B: *Escherichia coli* infection

Pyuria can occur in the absence of apparent bacterial infection (sterile pyuria), particularly in patients who have already taken antimicrobials (often due to self-medication). Patients with dysuria and frequency should be tested for atypical organisms such as *Chlamydia* or *Ureaplasma urealyticum* or for tuberculosis. Other causes of sterile pyuria include chronic interstitial nephritis (such as analgesic abuse nephropathy), uroepithelial tumour and nephrolithiasis. *E. coli* infection can be readily isolated and cultured from a mid-stream urine sample.

93 E: Coarctation of the aorta
There is an increased risk of cardiovascular morbidity and mortality in women with Turner's syndrome, presumably due to their risk of cardiovascular malformations, renal abnormalities and hypertension. The overall prevalence of cardiovascular malformations is 26%. Bicuspid aortic valve and coarctation of the aorta are the most common congenital abnormalities encountered in Turner's syndrome.

94 C: Vincristine
Alkylating agents exert their biological activity via their ability to covalently bind and crosslink a variety of macromolecules, including DNA, RNA and proteins. DNA crosslinking is the best studied and probably the most important biological action of these drugs. It results in impaired DNA replication and transcription, ultimately leading to either cell death or altered cellular function. Alkylating agents were first introduced as a treatment for autoimmune disease in the early 1950s and the group includes busulfan, melphalan and nitrogen mustard.

Vincristine is a vinca alkaloid and is a plant-derived cytotoxic agent whose mechanism of action involves anti-microtubule activity. It is not an alkylating agent.

95 D: Inhibition of ADH secretion
Angiotensin II is an oligopeptide of eight amino acids, formed from its original precursor, angiotensinogen, by a series of two enzymatic cleavages. Angiotensin II binds to its specific receptors and exerts its effects in the brain, kidney, adrenal gland, vascular wall and the heart. Its main functions include:

- Constriction of resistance vessels (via angiotensin II receptors), thereby increasing systemic vascular resistance and arterial pressure
- Action on the adrenal cortex to release aldosterone, which in turn acts on the kidneys to increase sodium and fluid retention
- Stimulation of the release of vasopressin (antidiuretic hormone, ADH) from the posterior pituitary which acts on the kidneys to increase fluid retention
- Stimulation of thirst centres within the brain

- Facilitation of noradrenaline (norepinephrine) release from sympathetic nerve endings and inhibition of its re-uptake by nerve endings, thereby enhancing sympathetic adrenergic function
- Stimulation of cardiac hypertrophy and vascular hypertrophy.

96 A: Adrenaline (epinephrine)

The adrenal glands are paired organs that functionally consist of three tissues under independent control – the outer cortex, the inner cortex and the medulla. The outer cortex is mainly controlled by the renin–angiotensin system, which regulates the release of aldosterone, which affects both sodium and potassium homeostasis. The inner cortex is mainly controlled by the corticotrophin-releasing hormone (CRH)–corticotrophin (ACTH) system, which regulates responses to stress via the actions of cortisol; it also produces adrenal androgens. The medulla is part of the sympathetic nervous system and produces adrenaline (epinephrine). Cells in the adrenal medulla synthesise and secrete noradrenaline (norepinephrine) and adrenaline (epinephrine). The ratio of these two catecholamines differs considerably among species: in humans, roughly 80% of the catecholamine output is adrenaline (epinephrine).

97 D: Inferolateral

The third (oculomotor), fourth (trochlear) and sixth (abducens) cranial nerves supply the muscles of the orbit. They enter the orbit through the superior orbital fissure. The fourth cranial nerve supplies the superior oblique muscle which rotates the eyeball in an inferolateral direction; the sixth cranial nerve supplies the lateral rectus muscle which abducts the eye; and the third cranial nerve supplies levator palpebrae superioris which elevates the eyelid, and the medial, superior, and inferior rectus muscles, which rotate the eyeball in the same direction. In third cranial nerve palsy, the actions of the muscles supplied by the fourth and sixth cranial nerves are unopposed.

98 E: Patients suspected of having Cushing's syndrome should undergo a dexamethasone suppression test

In renovascular hypertension a systolic–diastolic abdominal bruit that lateralises to one side is highly specific but identified in only 40% of cases (and therefore absent in many patients). Systolic bruits alone are more sensitive but less specific.

Causes of secondary hypertension other than primary aldosteronism include diuretic therapy, which may be surreptitious. Less common causes include Cushing's syndrome, certain forms of congenital adrenal hyperplasia, and rare renin-secreting tumours.

Hyperthyroidism is associated with increased cardiac contractility, increased cardiac output, and systolic hypertension. It also causes a reduction in systemic vascular resistance and diastolic pressure, resulting in widened pulse pressure.

Measurements of plasma or urine catecholamines and metabolites are diagnostic in 95% of patients with symptoms. Biochemical confirmation of the diagnosis should be followed by radiological evaluation to locate the tumour, not the other way around. About 10% of the tumours are extra-adrenal.

The diagnosis of hypercortisolism is usually established by demonstrating increased urinary cortisol excretion and, if necessary, impaired suppression of cortisol secretion during low-dose suppression.

99 C: Small bowel biopsy

The approximate sensitivity and specificity of the serum endomysial and antigliadin antibody tests is as follows:

- IgA endomysial antibodies – sensitivity 85–98%; specificity 97–100%
- IgA tissue transglutaminase antibodies – sensitivity 90–98%; specificity 95–97%
- IgA antigliadin antibodies – sensitivity 80–90%; specificity 85–95%
- IgG antigliadin antibodies – sensitivity 75–85%; specificity 75–90%

A positive IgA endomysial test is virtually diagnostic, but small bowel biopsy should still be considered to confirm gluten-sensitive enteropathy. The specificities of IgA and IgG antigliadin tests are lower and positive results have a low positive predictive value in low-risk populations.

100 E: Cognitive behavioural therapy

The diagnosis here is simple phobia, characterised by anxiety excessive to the perceived threat, and escape and avoidance conditioning. Although this may respond to antidepressants, the preferred treatment is cognitive behavioural therapy (CBT), using systematic desensitisation. The patient negotiates her goal (in this example this could be holding an unprotected needle) and identifies with the therapist successive stages of increasing exposure (usually about 8–12) to reach this goal. CBT may also involve 'homework' to maintain progress between appointments with the therapist.

PAPER TWO ANSWERS

101 B: Metabolic alkalosis

Three alcohols can produce potentially fatal intoxication: methanol, ethylene glycol and isopropyl alcohol (isopropanol). All can increase the anion gap, and the first two are typically associated with a potentially severe high-anion-gap metabolic acidosis.

With ethylene glycol (antifreeze solution) intoxication, the earliest findings are neurological abnormalities, ranging from drunkenness to coma. If untreated, these changes may be followed by cardiopulmonary symptoms (tachypnoea, pulmonary oedema) and then flank pain and renal failure, which may be accompanied by marked calcium oxalate crystalluria in the urine sediment. Urine examination by Wood's light (ultraviolet) may reveal fluorescence if the patient has ingested antifreeze solution, which is commonly adulterated with fluorescein dye. Fomepizole is now the antidote of choice in cases of methanol and ethylene glycol intoxication.

102 E: Ataxic nystagmus

Temporal lobe lesions cause receptive dysphasia and an upper homonymous quadrantanopia. Psychomotor epilepsy (complex partial seizures) is caused by medial temporal lobe-lesions. Manifestations include visual and auditory hallucinations, awareness of abnormal taste, feelings of fear, *déjà vu*, and depersonalisation and unfamiliarisation with surroundings.

Ataxic nystagmus is nystagmus greater in abducting eye, with impaired adduction, due to damage to the medial longitudinal fasciculus, causing internuclear ophthalmoplegia. The lesion lies within the pons.

103 E: Loperamide

Pharmacological agents are only an adjunct to treatment in IBS. Furthermore, the drug chosen varies depending on the patient's major symptoms. Diarrhoea-predominant IBS is therefore treated differently from constipation-predominant disease. For abdominal pain, consider antispasmodic (anticholinergic) medication, particularly when symptoms are exacerbated by meals, or a tricyclic antidepressant, particularly if pain is frequent or severe. For constipation, increased dietary fibre (25 g/day) is recommended for simple constipation, although evidence of its effectiveness in reducing pain is mixed. For diarrhoea, loperamide (2–4 mg, up to four times daily) can reduce loose stools, urgency and faecal soiling.

104   B: Giant cell arteritis

In giant cell arteritis (GCA) impaired vision is often an early manifestation of the disease. Affected patients typically note abrupt development of a partial field defect in one eye, which may progress to total blindness. If untreated, the second eye is likely to become affected within one to two weeks. It usually causes central retinal artery occlusion and, if undetected, the patient can develop severe, bilateral vision loss. Permanent visual loss may be partial or complete and may occur without warning; about 50% are unilateral and 50% are bilateral. Patients with central retinal artery occlusion over the age of 60 need an immediate erythrocyte sedimentation rate (ESR) to examine for the possibility of GCA. The universally accepted treatment for GCA is high-dose corticosteroid therapy. The major justification for the use of corticosteroids is the impending danger of blindness in untreated patients.

Papilloedema is generally not associated with visual loss. However, an enlarged blind spot and tunnel vision are recognised features of chronic papilloedema. In retinal vein occlusion the patient may be asymptomatic, but often will complain of sudden painless unilateral loss of vision and/or visual field. Ophthalmoscopically, there will be retinal oedema, superficial haemorrhages, disc swelling, cotton wool spots, and tortuous and dilated retinal veins. Migraine vasospasm might cause sudden unilateral visual loss. It is often associated with or followed by unilateral headache, unlike blindness in GCA which is often painless. In open angle glaucoma the blindness is often unilateral with a slow course.

105   B: Stop oxygen therapy immediately

The major danger facing patients who develop hypercapnia during treatment with oxygen is the abrupt removal of supplemental oxygen, causing the PaO_2 to fall to a level lower than when oxygen therapy was begun. In addition, the development of hypoxaemia in this setting is more rapid than the resolution of hypercapnia, and subsequent tissue hypoxia can potentially worsen the patient's acidaemia.

106   D: Valproate

The ultimate goal of treatment for women receiving antiepileptic drugs and oral contraceptives is to avoid unplanned pregnancies, while attaining optimal seizure control. Antiepileptic drugs affect many oral contraceptives. The metabolism of oral contraceptives is accelerated by any drug that increases liver microsomal enzyme activity (eg carbamazepine, phenytoin, phenobarbital, primidone, oxcarbazepine and topiramate). As a result, the contraceptive efficacy of an oral contraceptive is likely to be decreased in women taking these drugs. Valproate does not, and may even increase hormonal levels. Gabapentin, lamotrigine, tiagabine, and vigabatrin may also prove to be safe with oral contraceptives, but more research is needed.

107 B: Optic neuritis
Optic neuritis is the most common type of involvement of the visual pathways in patients with MS. It usually presents as acute or subacute unilateral eye pain that is accentuated by ocular movements. This is followed by a variable degree of visual loss (scotoma) affecting mainly central vision. A bilateral internuclear ophthalmoplegia (INO) is most suggestive of MS, but also can be observed with other intra-axial brainstem lesions, including brainstem glioma, or vascular lesions.

108 C: Interleukin-1 (IL-1)
Advances in research have identified specific cells and cell products (primarily cytokines) that may play distinct roles in RA activity. It has been well documented that in RA proinflammatory cytokines mediate synovial proliferation and articular tissue destruction. For these reasons, cytokines have become a target for therapy.

Cytokine-based therapies include agents which block proinflammatory cytokines (IL-1, IL-2, IL-6, IL-8, TNF-α, G-CSF, GM-CSF) and agents which augment anti-inflammatory cytokines (IL-4, IL-10, IL-11, IL-13, TGF-β, soluble TNF receptors, soluble IL-2 receptors).

109 B: Supraclavicular
Supraclavicular nodes are the most likely to be malignant and should always be investigated, even in children. Overall, the prevalence of malignancy is unknown, but rates of 54–85% have been seen in biopsy series reports. Abdominal and thoracic neoplasms are important primary sites that spread to the supraclavicular lymph nodes.

The incidence of palpable cervical lymph nodes, which are commonly appreciable throughout childhood, declines with age. The most common cause of cervical lymphadenopathy is infection, which in children is typically an acute and self-limited viral infection. While most cases resolve quickly, some conditions such as atypical mycobacteria, cat-scratch disease, toxoplasmosis and sarcoidosis can give rise to persistent lymphadenopathy for many months and may be confused with neoplasms. Axillary and epitrochlear lymph nodes drain the upper extremity which are commonly exposed to local infection and injury. Most axillary lymphadenopathy is non-specific or reactive. Inguinal lymphadenopathy is common, with nodes enlarged up to 1–2 cm in diameter in many healthy adults, particularly those who spend time barefoot outdoors. Benign reactive lymphadenopathy and infection are the most common causes. Inguinal lymphadenopathy is of low suspicion for malignancy.

110 C: Open biopsy

Open biopsy generally is the best diagnostic test because histological examination of intact tissue provides information about both the presence of abnormal cells (carcinoma, micro-organisms) and abnormal node architecture, which is necessary for the diagnosis of lymphomas. False-negative results occur when the wrong node is taken, which is not uncommon.

Incisional wedge biopsy might be helpful when full excision is not possible. It provides histological diagnosis but carries the inherent risk of missing the diagnosis when the malignant process is patchy and when necrotic tissue has replaced a large part of the gland. Fine-needle aspiration for cytology is most useful when searching for recurrence of cancer. Radiological tests can define the node size more precisely than physical examination, but add little to the diagnosis.

111 C: Retinal artery occlusion

The clinical picture is typical of central retinal artery occlusion. Patients with this condition present with a sudden, painless, unilateral loss of vision and/or visual field.

Ophthalmoscopically, you will see a pale, milky, oedematous retina with attenuated arterioles and a cherry-red macula if the entire central retinal artery is occluded. Embolism is usually caused by cholesterol emboli originating from the internal carotid arteries. Embolus from the heart is the most common cause of central retinal artery occlusion in patients younger than 40 years. Coagulopathies from sickle cell anaemia or antiphospholipid antibodies are common causes of central retinal artery occlusion in patients younger than 30 years.

112 C: Mobitz type II second-degree atrioventricular (AV) block

Digoxin toxicity is an important clinical problem and it may be potentially life-threatening. Factors that can increase the risk of digoxin intoxication include renal insufficiency, electrolyte abnormalities (hypokalaemia, hypomagnesaemia and hypercalcaemia), hypothyroidism and pulmonary disease. Almost any arrhythmia can be seen with digoxin toxicity. There are, however, some arrhythmias that are generally not induced by digoxin. Atrial flutter, atrial fibrillation, and Mobitz type II second-degree AV block are the least likely of all the arrhythmias to be caused by digoxin toxicity.

Bradyarrhythmias may be due to an excessive increase in vagal (parasympathetic) tone. First-degree block: some degree of PR lengthening may be expected with digoxin therapy. More marked widening of the PR interval to above 0.20 s suggests early digoxin toxicity. Second-degree block: with higher doses of digoxin, first-degree AV block may progress to second-degree block of the Mobitz type I (Wenckebach) variety. In contrast, Mobitz type II second-degree AV block is rarely induced by digoxin. Third-degree heart block: third-degree (complete) heart block and other types of AV dissociation may also occur with digoxin toxicity. AV junctional rhythms are frequently a sign of digoxin toxicity. The usual junctional escape rate is 30–50 bpm.

113 A: Atenolol

This is a case of myocardial infarction caused by cocaine use. The mechanism through which cocaine causes ischaemia and myocardial infarction seems to be complex and multifactorial. The main effect of cocaine is the inhibition of noradrenaline (norepinephrine) and dopamine re-uptake at the pre-synaptic level, causing their excessive accumulation in the meta-synaptic receptors. Cocaine therefore acts as a potent sympathomimetic agent. In the cardiovascular system it causes an increase of the heart rate, a rise in the arterial pressure and increased myocardial contractility. These three major haemodynamic changes increase myocardial oxygen demand. At the same time, by stimulating α-adrenergic receptors, it causes an intense spasm of the coronary arteries, particularly of the epicardiac arteries. Other effects of cocaine that further aggravate arterial spasm include increased endothelin production by the endothelium, which has been known to be a potent vasoconstrictive agent, and the reduction of nitric oxide production (a vasodilating agent). The increase in myocardial oxygen demand on the one hand and its reduced availability on the other are responsible for the myocardial ischaemia.

Another mechanism participating in the mechanism of infarction is the activation of platelets. The treatment of choice for the vasospasm is the administration of glyceryl trinitrate, verapamil or α-adrenergic receptor antagonists (fentolamine), while the use of β-adrenergic blockers is contraindicated as they usually aggravate the vasospasm. The administration of aspirin is also suggested for the inhibition of platelet agglutination. Benzodiazepines are useful because they reduce the heart rate and the arterial pressure. β-Adrenergic blockers should be avoided in the treatment of cocaine-induced myocardial ischaemia, which is best treated with nitrates and calcium-channel blockers.

114 C: ECT is effective treatment in certain patients with schizophrenia
Schizophrenia is a mental illness characterised by a multiplicity of symptoms affecting the most fundamental human attributes – cognition, emotion and perception. Monotherapy is preferred and polypharmacy is avoided as far as possible. Patients who have not responded to recommended antipsychotic medications should be considered for ECT. Usually the strategy would be to combine ECT with another antipsychotic treatment. ECT is effective for schizophrenic patients with affective or catatonic symptoms. Antidepressants should be considered for persistent depressive symptoms and should be prescribed with an antipsychotic to prevent worsening of psychosis. Post-psychotic ('residual' or secondary) depressive symptoms have been shown to respond to antidepressant treatment. Because of the potentially fatal idiosyncratic side effect of agranulocytosis, patients on clozapine should have their full blood count monitored weekly for the first 18 weeks and monthly thereafter. Clozapine does not cause any liver abnormality that requires regular monitoring of liver function. The use of both typical and atypical antipsychotic drugs is associated with an increased risk of neuroleptic malignant syndrome.

115 D: The patient's brothers and sisters are probably at a higher risk than his children
Hereditary haemochromatosis is a genetic iron overload disorder, caused by excessive unregulated absorption of iron. It is associated with homozygosity for mutations in the haemochromatosis (*HFE*) gene on the short arm of chromosome 6. Most patients have a substitution of tyrosine for cysteine in amino acid number 282 (C282Y). Hereditary haemochromatosis is inherited as an autosomal recessive trait.

Screening of other family members (or populations) may allow diagnosis at an early stage, before there has been irreversible organ damage. Accordingly, there is general agreement that first-degree relatives of patients with hereditary haemochromatosis should be screened for the disease. In contrast, population screening for the disease remains a topic of debate. If the proband is homozygous for C282Y mutation, the spouse undergoes genetic testing to determine whether they are also a carrier for a mutation. If the spouse is heterozygous for the C282Y the children undergo genetic testing. Screening of young children of patients with haemochromatosis does not need to be performed if the spouse is tested and does not have the C282Y mutation. The optimal timing for screening family members is between the ages of 18 and 30. As in any autosomal recessive disease, siblings are generally at a higher risk of having the disease than the children.

116   C: Multiple myeloma

In multiple myeloma bone pain and lytic bone lesions are very common, caused by tumour expansion and by activation of osteoclasts by myeloma cell secretion of osteoclast activation factors. Interleukin-6 may play an important role in osteoclast activation and bone reabsorption. Because of low bone density pathological fractures are common. Another common problem is hypercalcaemia which may lead to renal changes and neurological symptoms if not treated. It is caused by increased bone resorption.

Osteomalacia and osteoporosis are associated with reduced bone density but not with hypercalcaemia. On the other hand, sarcoidosis is often associated with hypercalcaemia and arthropathy but does not lead to lytic bone lesions. Paget's disease of the bone is characterised by somewhat thicker than normal bones which have a 'coarse' pattern of bone trabeculae. This appearance results from an increased rate of bone turnover. Paget's disease results in bones that are somewhat more brittle than normal bones. Calcium levels are typically normal unless there is history of recent fracture or prolonged bedrest.

117   C: Carcinoma of the stomach

Acanthosis nigricans (AN) is asymptomatic, brown-black eruptions with a velvety texture. Pedunculated skin tags are often present. The most common sites are the axillae, neck and groin. If the patient is obese, the eruption may clear with weight loss or correction of the underlying endocrine disorder. Local treatment is not effective. AN is usually classified into two types: a benign form, not associated with malignancy, and a malignant form. Patients with the malignant form of AN tend to be thin and aged over 40, and their eruption is of recent origin. The most common malignancy associated with malignant AN is abdominal adenocarcinoma, especially of the stomach.

Most patients with the benign form are obese. Some have an endocrinopathy, such as diabetes mellitus, especially of the insulin-resistant type; pituitary or adrenal adenomas; Cushing's syndrome; acromegaly; an intake of diethylstilbestrol; or the Stein–Leventhal syndrome (polycystic ovary disease). Other causes include chronic hepatitis and ingestion of large doses of niacin.

118 A: Hepatitis C virus (HCV)

The clinical picture and immunology profile is compatible with the diagnosis of essential mixed cryoglobulinaemia (EMC). This condition results in the deposition of circulating immune complexes in small- to medium-sized blood vessels. Patients with EMC usually present with rash, arthralgias and weakness. A review of the literature reveals that hepatitis C can be found in 95% of all patients with EMC. Several investigators have suggested that hepatitis C may have a causative role in EMC. Anti-HCV antibodies can be detected in the vessel walls of skin biopsy specimens taken from patients with EMC and chronic vasculitis. Interferon therapy has been shown to reduce the cryocrit and lead to symptomatic improvement of both rash and joint pains. The response is short-lived, however, because symptoms almost universally reappear on cessation of therapy.

119 B: Acoustic neuroma

An acoustic neuroma (sometimes also called a 'neurinoma' or 'vestibular schwannoma') is a benign growth that arises from the eighth cranial (vestibulocochlear) nerve. Once the tumour fully occupies the internal auditory canal, it often begins to erode the walls of the canal and enlarges it, which can be detected on X-rays or by MRI. As the tumour slowly enlarges towards the brain, it protrudes from the internal auditory canal into the cerebellopontine angle.

Meningioma may originate from the meninges over the cerebral hemisphere and presents with seizures, focal neurological deficits or headaches. Falx and parasagittal meningiomas may result in bilateral leg weakness. Medulloblastomas demonstrate a bimodal age distribution, with a larger peak at 2–8 years and a smaller peak at 20–30 years. Exclusively cerebellar, medulloblastomas typically arise from the cerebellar vermis and the roof of the fourth ventricle in the younger age group and, less commonly, from the cerebellar hemisphere in the older age group. Cholesteatoma may cause erosion of the ossicles or bones behind the eardrum and leads to a conductive hearing loss. The hallmark symptom of cholesteatoma is painless otorrhoea. It does not extend to the cerebellopontine angle.

120 A: The use of a needle to obtain the female mite from the skin lesion

Scabies is an intensely pruritic and highly contagious infestation of the skin caused by a mite affecting humans and other animals. *Sarcoptes scabiei* var *hominis* is the cause of human scabies. It lives its entire life on the human host. Identifying the mite and its eggs or faeces in skin scrapings from involved sites confirms the diagnosis of scabies. Samples are best obtained from a non-excoriated papule or burrow. A drop of oil is placed on top of the lesion or directly on a no. 15 scalpel blade, which is used to scrape a burrow vigorously (try to avoid causing bleeding). Transfer the material collected from the skin onto a glass slide and examine with 40× microscopic magnification to try and identify the mite, its eggs, or faeces.

121 D: Congestive cardiac failure

A marked inspiratory decrease in arterial pressure, exceeding 20 mmHg, is called 'pulsus paradoxus'. In contrast to the normal situation, this is easily detectable by palpation, although it should be evaluated with a sphygmomanometer. When the cuff pressure is slowly released the systolic pressure at expiration is first noted. With further slow deflation of the cuff, the systolic pressure during inspiration can also be detected. The difference between the pressures noted during expiration and inspiration is the magnitude of the pulsus paradoxus. Pulsus paradoxus is an important physical finding in cardiac tamponade. In addition to tamponade, pulsus paradoxus can occur in chronic obstructive pulmonary disease, hypovolaemic shock and, infrequently, in constrictive pericarditis and restrictive cardiomyopathy.

122 B: Paul–Bunnell test

Causes of reactive lymphocytosis may be: β-streptococci, cytomegalovirus, drugs, Epstein–Barr virus (EBV), syphilis, toxoplasmosis, vaccination, and viral hepatitis. The symptoms of fever, pharyngitis, and lymphadenopathy are typical of acute EBV infection (infectious mononucleosis). The most useful laboratory test to diagnose infectious mononucleosis is the serological test for heterophil antibodies (Paul–Bunnell test).

123   C: Marfan's syndrome

The role of genetic factors in the pathogenesis of intracranial aneurysm formation is supported by studies which have found an increased risk in patients with some known hereditary syndromes and by the occurrence of aneurysms in families. A known hereditary syndrome is often present when aneurysms are diagnosed in more than one family member. Heritable disorders associated with the presence of intracranial aneurysm include connective tissue diseases, such as Ehlers–Danlos syndrome and pseudoxanthoma elasticum (but probably not Marfan's syndrome) and autosomal dominant polycystic kidney disease. Other factors that may increase the risk of aneurysmal subarachnoid haemorrhage include cigarette smoking, hypertension, oestrogen deficiency, and moderate to high alcohol consumption. Patients with coarctation of the aorta are also at increased risk of aneurysm formation.

124   B: Serum cholesterol

On initial evaluation it is critical to determine if primary skin lesions are present. In the absence of primary skin lesions, pruritus can be the presenting symptom in a wide range of systemic diseases. Chronic renal failure is the systemic disease most commonly linked with generalised pruritus. Pruritus occurs in up to 90% of haemodialysis patients. Biliary diseases, including intrahepatic and extrahepatic cholestasis, drug-induced cholestasis and primary biliary cirrhosis, also commonly result in generalised itching. Endocrine diseases that are accompanied by pruritus include diabetes mellitus, hyperthyroidism and hypothyroidism. Haematological causes include iron deficiency anaemia, polycythaemia rubravera and plasma cell dyscrasias.

125   C: Move patient to a well lit single room

This patient has developed a delirium (acute confusional state) probably secondary to pneumonia. Other common causes in older people include urinary tract infections, medication (especially analgesics), constipation, pain, hypoxia and alcohol withdrawal! Delirium is commonly missed on medical wards. The management includes identifying and treating the cause. Disturbed patients may require small doses of antipsychotic medication although benzodiazepines should be used as a last resort. In a florid presentation described above, moving the patient to a well-lit single room with 1:1 observation with a familiar experienced nurse may help to reduce disorientation and paranoid beliefs.

126　D: Serum transferrin saturation (TS)

High transferrin saturation is the earliest evidence of haemochromatosis. It is the initial test of choice. Measuring the transferrin saturation (TS = serum iron divided by total iron-binding capacity) is the most effective and inexpensive screening test for iron overload. Blood should be drawn in the fasting state, because iron levels may increase after a meal. It is suggested that if TS is equal to or higher than 45%, the test should be repeated, together with serum ferritin determination. If TS (with or without high ferritin) is elevated, *HFE* genes should be determined, particularly in patients of Northern European origin. Liver biopsy is necessary if iron overload syndrome is suspected on the basis of a high TS and elevated ferritin level. Ferritin levels are less sensitive than transferrin saturation in screening tests for haemochromatosis. Ferritin concentration can be high in other conditions, such as infections, inflammations and liver disease. Measuring serum iron or haemoglobin has no value in the diagnosis.

127　D: Adrenal failure

The prothrombin time assesses the extrinsic pathway of the blood coagulation cascade. In jaundiced patients and patients with malabsorption the absorption of fat-soluble vitamins, including vitamin K, is reduced. Vitamin K is necessary for the synthesis of clotting factors II, VII, IX and XI. Warfarin is a vitamin K antagonist. Heparin potentiates the activity of antithrombin III and has no effect on the external pathway or prothrombin time.

128　E: Group B vaccine is far more effective than group A or C vaccines

At least 13 serogroups have been described: A, B, C, D, E, H, I, K, L, W135, X, Y and Z. Serogroups B and C have caused most cases of meningococcal meningitis.

Currently, penicillin is the drug of choice for the treatment of meningococcal meningitis and septicaemia. Person-to-person transmission can be interrupted by chemoprophylaxis, which eradicates the asymptomatic nasopharyngeal carrier state. Rifampin, quinolones, and ceftriaxone are the antimicrobials used to eradicate meningococci from the nasopharynx. Vaccination is used for close contacts of patients with meningococcal disease due to A, C, Y, or W135 serogroups to prevent secondary cases. No effective vaccine exists to protect individuals from meningococcal meningitis caused by serogroup B.

129 C: The reticulocyte count is low in relation to the degree of anaemia

The history and the blood picture are suggestive of iron deficiency anaemia.

In the first stage, iron stores can be totally depleted without causing anaemia. The storage iron pool consists primarily of ferritin and haemosiderin-bound iron within the monocyte-macrophage system, chiefly in bone marrow, liver and spleen. Further loss of iron results in anaemia, which is initially normocytic with a normal absolute reticulocyte count. More profound deficiency results in the classical hypochromia and microcytosis of iron-deficient erythropoiesis. The serum iron is low and the total iron-binding capacity (TIBC) is elevated (> 72 μmol/l), resulting in a low transferrin saturation. The plasma ferritin concentration is usually reduced. The platelet counts are often elevated in response to anaemia and/or the underlying blood loss.

Gastrointestinal bleeding is the commonest cause of iron deficiency anaemia in men. The patient responded briskly to oral iron therapy with a reticulocytosis, followed by elevations in the haemoglobin concentration and haematocrit. In contrast to haemolytic anaemia, iron is not available to produce more RBCs (reticulocytes) to match the tissue demands for carrying the required oxygen and nutrients to maintain viability.

130 C: Tetracycline

Tetracycline treats susceptible bacterial infections of both Gram-positive and Gram-negative organisms, as well as infections caused by *Mycoplasma, Chlamydia* and *Rickettsia* organisms. It inhibits bacterial protein synthesis by binding with the 30S subunit and possibly the 50S ribosomal subunit of susceptible bacteria. It is as effective as erythromycin and other macrolides in the treatment of *Mycoplasma pneumoniae* infection.

131 B: Posterior communicating artery aneurysm

Diplopia and sluggish or absent reaction to light is most likely to be due to compression injury to the oculomotor nerve (third cranial nerve). Pupillary dilatation and a sluggish or absent reaction to light results from involvement of parasympathetic fibres that originate in the Edinger–Westphal subnucleus of the third cranial nerve complex. They are situated very superficially within the nerve trunk and hence are damaged by compression injury, most often seen with posterior communicating artery aneurysm. A third nerve palsy with pupillary sparing is often called a 'medical' third nerve palsy and often has an ischaemic or diabetic cause. The ischaemic injury will damage the inner tissues of the nerve trunk and spare the superficial parasympathetic fibres which have an alternative blood supply.

The pupil is never involved in myasthenia gravis or other ocular myopathy although these patients typically present with diplopia. Internuclear ophthalmoplegia (INO) is the most common ocular motility dysfunction in multiple sclerosis. The patient will manifest an adduction deficit on the involved side and a nystagmus of the fellow eye in extreme abduction. It is caused by lesions through the medial longitudinal fasciculus in the pons. The pupil is not involved.

132 B: Pulmonary tuberculosis

Airborne transmission occurs when bacteria or viruses travel on dust particles or on small respiratory droplets that may become aerosolised when people sneeze, cough, laugh or exhale. They hang in the air much like invisible smoke. They can travel on air currents over considerable distances. These droplets are loaded with infectious particles. The amount of exposure necessary varies from disease to disease. With chickenpox, a child could easily catch it from another aisle in a supermarket. With tuberculosis, closer contact and less air circulation are often needed. Many common infections can spread by airborne transmission, at least in some cases, including anthrax (inhalational), chickenpox, influenza, measles, pertussis (whooping cough), smallpox and tuberculosis.

133 C: Typhoid fever

Patients who are suffering from contagious infections are often nursed in isolation using a procedure known as barrier nursing. These techniques have developed to protect the hospital environment from contamination with dangerous pathogens. Anything that comes into direct contact with the patient is considered infective and must be sterilised before being returned to general use. If this proves impossible then the item must be incinerated before disposal. Personnel attending the infectious patient wear special protective clothing, masks and gloves. Typhoid fever is caused by an infection with the bacterium *Salmonella typhi*, which is only found in humans. Typhoid germs are passed in the faeces and, to some extent, the urine of infected people. The germs are spread by eating or drinking water or foods contaminated by faeces from the infected individual. In legionellosis there is no risk of disease spread from human to human.

134 A: Fever
Thoracentesis is most frequently performed to determine the cause of a pleural effusion (ie diagnostic). However, thoracentesis is sometimes performed to relieve respiratory insufficiency caused by a large pleural effusion (ie therapeutic). The indication for diagnostic thoracentesis is a new finding of a pleural effusion. Observation, in lieu of diagnostic thoracentesis, may be warranted in uncomplicated congestive heart failure where the clinical diagnosis is usually secure. Pleural effusions characteristically accumulate in the right hemithorax and later bilaterally. Lymphatic drainage is greatly enhanced but cannot overcome the increase in lung water. In most cases diuretics will be the first line of treatment. A dramatic response with reduction of pleural and peripheral fluid collections is anticipated. However, the emergence of signs of infections such as fever, rigors and pleuritic chest pain, might suggest an infective process such as empyema and diagnostic thoracentesis would therefore be essential to secure the diagnosis and prompt the use of appropriate antibiotics.

135 A: Papillitis
'Papillitis' or anterior optic neuritis is a general term implying inflammation of the optic nerve, but also embraces degeneration or demyelination of the optic nerve. It is indistinguishable ophthalmoscopically from papilloedema. Central scotomata are the most common visual field defect. Unlike papilloedema, papillitis is accompanied by a dramatic decrease in visual acuity, and pain in the eye when it is moved. The disease process is usually unilateral. Causes of papillitis include multiple sclerosis, viral illness, temporal arteritis and other kinds of inflammation of the arteries (vasculitis), and poisoning by chemicals such as lead and methanol.

136 C: Spinal accessory nerve
The spinal accessory nerve originates from neuronal cell bodies located in the cervical spinal cord and caudal medulla. Most are located in the spinal cord and ascend through the foramen magnum and exit the cranium through the jugular foramen. They are branchiomotor in function and innervate the sternocleidomastoid and trapezius muscles in the neck and back. Nerve injuries may result from lymph node biopsies or other surgical procedures in the neck region or occasionally after other trauma. Spinal accessory nerve injury can cause a drooping shoulder, muscle atrophy, and weakened or limited elevation or abduction of the arm/shoulder. It

can also cause shoulder pain and winging of the upper border of the scapula with lateral abduction of the shoulder.

In axillary nerve injury the most common complaint is shoulder weakness, especially when lifting the arm out from the side of the body. Sometimes the shoulder can still go through a full range of motion, although with less power. Within weeks of the injury, the muscle bulk over the outside of the shoulder will become noticeably smaller. Loss of sensation over the skin of the outer border of the shoulder may be noticed. The scapula is not affected.

137 B: Dermatitis herpetiformis

Coeliac disease is associated with a number of skin disorders, of which dermatitis herpetiformis is the most common. Dermatitis herpetiformis is characterised by an itchy papular vesicular eruption, usually located symmetrically on the elbows, knees, buttocks, sacrum, face, neck, trunk and occasionally within the mouth. The predominant symptoms are itching and burning that are rapidly relieved by rupture of the blisters.

138 A: *Streptococcus bovis* is part of the normal oral flora

Streptococcus bovis is a Gram-positive coccus. The most common manifestations of *S. bovis* infection are bacteraemia and infective endocarditis. The organism is usually susceptible to penicillin, and infection generally responds to the same treatment regimens prescribed for infections due to *S. viridans*. In view of the association between *S. bovis* bacteraemia or infective endocarditis with colonic neoplasia, strong recommendations have been made that all adult patients with *S. bovis* bacteraemia undergo an aggressive diagnostic evaluation to search for colonic malignancy. The organism is not generally considered to be part of the normal oral flora although bacteria described as *S. bovis* have been identified in cultures from the gums or throat in small numbers of individuals.

139 A: This may result from dietary carbohydrate intolerance

In coeliac disease (also called gluten enteropathy and non-tropical sprue) gliadine, wheat, barley, rye, and (to a minor degree) oats trigger malabsorption. The primary findings are mucosal inflammation, crypt hyperplasia and villous atrophy. The coeliac lesion is confined in the proximal small intestine. Serum IgA endomysial antibody testing has the highest diagnostic accuracy. It is moderately sensitive and highly specific for gluten-sensitive enteropathy. Coeliac disease is associated with an increased incidence of cancer. The most common malignancy is lymphoma (18%). Coeliac disease is frequently associated with dermatitis herpetiformis. This condition is characterised by pruritic papulovesicles over the external surfaces of the extremities and on the trunk. The cornerstone of treating coeliac disease is the complete elimination of gluten from the diet.

140 D: Cell-mediated delayed response

Allergic contact dermatitis occurs when contact with a particular substance elicits a delayed (type IV) hypersensitivity reaction. Anyone with normal cell-mediated immunity can develop allergic contact dermatitis and the ability to respond to certain antigens is probably genetically determined. Commonly identified triggers in this condition include nickel in jewellery (eg earrings) and fragrances.

141 E: Constrictive pericarditis

A transudate has a low protein concentration (< 25 g/l) and can result from a low serum protein concentration, high central venous pressure or portal hypertension. An exudate has a high protein concentration (> 25 g/l). Tuberculous peritonitis, peritoneal malignancy, Budd–Chiari syndrome, pancreatic ascites, chylous ascites and Meigs' syndrome can all give rise to an exudative ascites.

142 A: Induced sputum analysis

Pneumocystis carinii pneumonia (PCP) is the most likely diagnosis in this case. Gallium-67 citrate scanning is a highly sensitive test in patients with PCP, demonstrating intense, diffuse bilateral uptake. However, its role is limited by lack of specificity, its high cost, and a two-day delay in obtaining final results. Definitive diagnosis of PCP requires documentation of the organism in respiratory specimens. Conventional stains such as toluidine blue O, Grocott's methenamine silver or Giemsa can be used to identify the organism. The most rapid and least invasive method of diagnosing PCP is by analysis of sputum induced by the inhalation of hypertonic saline. While the specificity of this method approaches 100%, the sensitivity ranges from 55–92%. This variability is related to the prevalence of PCP in the patient population, the skill of the team inducing the sputum, and the expertise of the laboratory in processing and interpreting the specimen. If sputum induction is non-diagnostic or cannot be performed (eg the patient cannot co-operate, is too dyspnoeic or has an altered mental state), then fiberoptic bronchoscopy with bronchoalveolar lavage is recommended, with or without transbronchial biopsy. Although lung biopsy, either by thoracotomy or by video-assisted thoracoscopic surgery, can be performed with an assurance of 100% sensitivity and specificity for the diagnosis of PCP, it is used very infrequently because of its cost and invasiveness.

143 D: Diabetic dermopathy
Nearly one-third of diabetic patients have some type of dermatological manifestation. This patient's rash is typical of diabetic dermopathy. It is the most common skin rash in diabetes mellitus and occurs in 40% of patients. Histologically, thickened superficial blood vessels, extravasation of erythrocytes and a mild lymphocytic infiltrate are often noted. The extravasated erythrocytes leave haemosiderin deposits, which provide the brownish hyperpigmentation. The lesions of diabetic dermopathy resolve spontaneously, leaving scars behind.

Necrobiosis lipoidica diabeticorum is also seen on the pretibial region of the lower extremities but the lesions are different and described as well-circumscribed erythematous plaques with a depressed, waxy telangiectatic centre. One-third of lesions may progress to ulcers. Scleroedema diabeticorum is an extensive non-pitting induration and thickening of the skin involving the posterior neck, upper part of the back, and the upper extremities, including the hands. Eruptive xanthomas in the context of diabetes mellitus are associated with hyperlipidaemic and hyperglycaemic states. The lesions are described as waxy yellow papules surrounded by an erythematous rim and usually occur on the extensor surfaces and in the popliteal region. Acanthosis nigricans is a disorder characterised by a velvety, light-brown to black hyperpigmented cutaneous thickening, usually on the back, the sides of the neck, the axillae and flexural surfaces.

144 B: Encapsulated bacteria
In patients who have HIV, the most common cause of chest infection is actually the group of encapsulated organisms, such as *Streptococcus pneumoniae* and *Haemophilus influenzae*. The most frequent opportunistic infection in these patients is with *Pneumocystis carinii*. Other important pulmonary infections include mycobacterial disease (typical and atypical), viral infections (eg cytomegalovirus), and fungal infections (eg histoplasmosis).

145 A: Ischaemic cerebral infarction is responsible for 80% of strokes
Approximately 80% of strokes are due to ischaemic cerebral infarction and 20% to brain haemorrhage. The proximal internal carotid artery and the carotid bifurcation are most frequently

involved. No surgical treatment has been proved to be of benefit for preventing a subsequent stroke in patients with complete carotid artery occlusion. However, contralateral carotid endarterectomy in patients with a symptomatic occlusion induces cerebral haemodynamic improvement on the side of surgery and on the side of the occlusion.

A bruit alone is a poor predictor of underlying carotid stenosis and for the subsequent development of stroke in asymptomatic patients. The number of patients with asymptomatic bruits who go on to have a stroke is small. Carotid bruits may be a better indicator of atherosclerotic disease in general than as a predictor of stroke. Most thrombotic and embolic strokes related to carotid atherosclerosis occur in older patients. Cardiac-origin embolism is also common in young people who are known to have heart disease.

146 E: Bladder carcinoma

Serum α-fetoprotein is a fetal serum protein produced by the yolk sac and liver. Increased serum levels in adults are seen in tumours (hepatocellular carcinoma, neuroblastomas and teratoma) and acute hepatitis and colitis. In patients with tumours, serum levels often correlate with tumour size. Resection is usually associated with a fall in serum levels. Serum levels are useful in assessing response to treatment.

147 D: Coxsackievirus B

Myocarditis is an uncommon disease that is characterised by inflammation of the heart. Subsequent myocardial destruction often leads to a dilated cardiomyopathy.

Viral myocarditis is by far the most common single cause in the US and Europe. The enterovirus group, with coxsackievirus B, may account for as many as 50% of cases. Other viruses implicated in myocarditis include influenza, echovirus, herpes simplex, varicella, hepatitis, Epstein–Barr and cytomegalovirus.

148 A: Spearman correlation

The number of consultations and the skills score are both integer variables taking a reasonable range of values. Note, they cannot be assumed to follow a continuous Normal distribution.

A is correct because it is a valid way to determine an association between two non-Normal measures.

B is not appropriate because although the simple chi-square test measures the association between two (categorical) variables, it does not take account of the ordering of the categories and requires there to be a reasonable number of subjects in each category.

C is inappropriate because the Mann–Whitney U-test is used to compare two groups w.r.t. a non-Normal variable, and hence requires one variable to be binary (two-category) and one variable to be a non-Normal measure. The skills score could be dichotomised into two categories, but the choice of a suitable cut-off score (to define high/low) would have to be justified and this strategy would also result in a loss of information for the skills score (ie. the full range of score would not be used in the analysis) leading to a less efficient test.

D is inappropriate because the data are not Normally distributed and a comparison of two paired groups is not required.

E is inappropriate because the data are not binary (two-category) and a comparison of two paired groups is not required.

149 E: Approximately 1–2% per year progress to carcinoma

Up to 50% of neonates have colonising *C. difficile* in their intestines but also an inherent protection against toxin A. Once the normal intestinal flora is established, *C. difficile* is not as prevalent, found in the faeces of only 3% of normal adults. If normal intestinal flora is altered, colonisation by toxigenic *C. difficile* can occur. Most responsible for the alteration of the normal intestinal flora and decreased resistance to *C. difficile* is the use of antibiotics, especially clindamycin. Other antibiotics associated with *C. difficile* infection include the amino penicillins, second- and third-generation cephalosporins and clarithromycin.

Sigmoidoscopy shows characteristic pseudomembranes surrounded by normal-looking mucosa. Because *C. difficile* may be a normal bowel organism (especially in children), simply culturing the organism does not mean that diarrhoea is caused by *C. difficile*. Cytotoxic assays are considered the standard criterion for laboratory diagnosis. Stool filtrate is mixed with mammalian tissue-culture cell lines and observed for cytopathic effect. Toxin can also be detected by latex agglutination, immunobinding assay, or ELISA. *C. difficile* infection and pseudomembranous colitis do not progress to carcinoma.

150 E: Spirometry

Full blood count, arterial blood gases, prothrombin time, partial thromboplastin time, sputum for Gram stain, culture and cytology, and urinalysis might be helpful. A recent chest X-ray to evaluate any obvious abnormalities is mandatory. Spirometry is not usually very helpful in the acute setting.

151 B: Colorectal cancer
Any tumour may involve bone. The most common include metastatic cancer of the breast, lung, prostate, thyroid and multiple myeloma. Common sites of bony metastasis are the vertebral column, skull, humerus, ribs, pelvis and femur. For colorectal cancer the most common metastatic sites are the regional lymph nodes, liver, lungs and peritoneum, and bone metastasis is relatively rare.

152 D: Bupropion hydrochloride
The serotonin re-uptake inhibitors (SSRIs) and venlafaxine are now known to occasionally cause significant changes in sexual response because of increased serotonin activity at the 5-HT$_2$ receptor site. Some patients complain of loss of libido and responsiveness, while others experience delayed time to orgasm. Mirtazapine and nefazodone are less likely than other antidepressants to cause sexual side effects because of their properties of 5-HT$_2$ antagonism. Also, bupropion has no direct serotoninergic activity and is not generally associated with such problems. One clinical report showed that using a low dose of bupropion along with an SSRI may obviate the serotoninergic sexual side effects.

153 C: Thrombus superimposed on pre-existing atherosclerotic plaque
As with all types of myocardial injury, Q-wave infarction is initiated in most instances by a thrombus superimposed on pre-existing atherosclerotic plaque, plus some degree of associated local vasoconstriction. In most cases coronary occlusion is sustained in Q-wave infarction, while in non-Q-wave infarction early spontaneous re-perfusion occurs. The sustained total occlusion results in extensive myocardial necrosis unless coronary flow can be restored early in the course of the event.

154 D: Continue with metformin and add glipizide
Initial therapy with an oral agent usually fails to control the blood glucose indefinitely. In fact, only one-third of patients maintained an Hb A$_{1c}$ level under 7% after six years of monotherapy. Therefore, a second oral agent of a different class is commonly added when glucose control begins to deteriorate. For glucose reduction, the combination of an insulin secretagogue (glipizide) and metformin produces a greater effect. Combinations of three oral agents are becoming increasingly popular for use before a patient's transition to insulin therapy. Thiazolidinediones, like metformin, improve insulin sensitivity. They can be substituted for metformin, especially

in patients with renal insufficiency or metformin intolerance. The response rate may be slightly less than that achieved with metformin in unselected patients with type 2 diabetes. The primary focus of any treatment strategy is reaching a target Hb A_{1c} level of 7% or less. When the initial Hb A_{1c} value exceeds 9%, a single agent is unlikely to accomplish this goal and in such cases a second agent is required.

155 B: Lymphoma
Of particular concern is the increased frequency of non-Hodgkin's lymphoma (about a 40-fold increase in relative risk) in patients with Sjögren's syndrome. There is a particular increase in the frequency of lymphoma involving the lymph nodes of the neck. In patients with persistent swelling of the parotid or submandibular glands imaging studies should be performed to look for associated adenopathy. The finding of persistent regional lymphadenopathy should lead to consideration of biopsy for lymphoma.

156 C: Communication may be possible with blinking eye movements
In persistent vegetative state the individual loses the higher cerebral powers but the functions of the brainstem, such as respiration (breathing) and circulation, remain relatively intact. Patients are completely paralysed but spontaneous movements may occur and the eyes may open in response to external stimuli. However, the patient does not speak, communicate or obey commands. The locked-in syndrome has some similarities to PVS as the person is almost completely paralysed. However, locked-in patients can often move their eyes purposefully, showing that they are conscious and aware of their environment. They can communicate with those around them. Tragically, they are otherwise unable to move.

Clinical features of PVS include:

- Spontaneous respiration
- No life-support machinery required
- Body functions normally
- Sleep/wake cycles are preserved
- Swallowing occurs, but not safely or sufficiently (hence tube feeding)
- No intellectual activity and no communication
- No rational responses
- No sentience
- No cognitive function.

Head injury and cerebral anoxia are the most common causes of PVS.

157 B: Volume overload
Hypertension is present in approximately 80–85% of patients with chronic renal failure. The prevalence of hypertension increases linearly as the glomerular filtration rate falls. Sodium and water retention with volume overload is the most important mechanism in hypertension complicating chronic renal failure, even though the degree of extracellular volume expansion may be insufficient to induce oedema. All the other options are factors that may contribute to some extent in individual patients.

158 A: Drug-induced systemic lupus erythematosus (SLE)
Drug-induced SLE is a syndrome that resembles mild idiopathic SLE and commonly presents after exposure to an offending drug as arthralgia or arthritis, myalgia and serositis. Extra-articular features include lethargy, myalgia, Raynaud's phenomenon, abdominal pain and a characteristic butterfly rash. Other systemic features include fever, hepatomegaly, splenomegaly, skin eruption, and the presence of antinuclear antibodies (ANA). The first case of drug-induced SLE was recognised in 1945. The classic drugs causing drug-induced SLE are hydralazine and procainamide, but because these drugs are now less commonly used, reports of new offending drugs have surfaced in the past few years. One of the drugs most recently implicated in drug-induced SLE is minocycline, a tetracycline derivative most commonly used to treat inflammatory acne. Symptoms usually resolve a few weeks after discontinuation of minocycline. Although the female-to-male ratio in idiopathic SLE is 9:1, males are equally as likely as females to develop drug-induced SLE.

159 B: Barium swallow
This patient suffers with dysphagia, which usually indicates some disorder of the oesophagus. Patients with scleroderma suffer with motility disorder in more than 90% of cases. Barium swallow can identify anatomical causes of dysphagia and some motor disorders, and can be better than endoscopy in diagnosing extrinsic compression. If barium swallow is normal, manometry might be helpful to assess motility disorders associated with scleroderma.

Endoscopy is usually the test of choice for obstruction, especially acute obstruction (eg food impaction), or if gastro-oesophageal reflux disease is suspected. Endoscopy offers the added advantage of obtaining biopsies, useful in diagnosing oesophagitis.

160 D: The most effective treatment is continuous positive airway pressure

The history and clinical examination might help to identify cases of this disorder, but reliable diagnosis is usually based on objective tests. A nocturnal polysomnogram performed in a sleep laboratory is the diagnostic procedure of choice. The test continuously records the electrical potentials of the brain and heart, eye movements, muscle activity, respiratory effort, airflow, oxygen saturation and leg movements throughout the night. The most common symptoms of OSAS are snoring and excessive daytime sleepiness. On awakening patients do not feel refreshed and often find it difficult to get out of bed. Some feel mentally dull, groggy, confused or disoriented. Daytime sleepiness is initially manifest during boring, sedentary situations in the afternoon or evening but later in the disease course patients may describe difficulty remaining awake during meetings after lunch or while driving or reading. Systemic hypertension, cardiac arrhythmias, peripheral neuropathy and gastro-oesophageal reflux are all recognised complications associated with OSAS. There is evidence for increased incidence of renal failure in patients with OSAS. The treatment of choice is continuous positive airway pressure (CPAP) applied through a nasal mask or nasal 'pillows', both of which function as an 'air splint' to maintain positive intraluminal pressure in the upper airway.

161 E: Immunoglobulin replacement is the definitive treatment for common variable immunodeficiency

This patient is clearly suffering from an immunoglobulin deficiency disorder rather than cellular immunity (T-cell) defects. Immunoglobulin deficiency disorders are associated with recurrent sino-pulmonary bacterial infections and sepsis involving encapsulated organisms. Sinusitis, otitis, bronchitis, pneumonia and bronchiectasis may be seen. Examples include common variable immunodeficiency and hyper-IgM syndrome.

Intravenous immunoglobulin replacement is the definitive treatment of primary immunoglobulin deficiency states. However, in selective IgA deficiency, blood products and intravenous immunoglobulin are contraindicated because of a high risk of anaphylactic events. Purified protein derivative is used to evaluate delayed-type hypersensitivity. All live viral vaccines are contraindicated in patients with impaired cell-mediated immunity. Patients with chronic granulomatous disease have phagocytic dysfunction that involves defects in intracellular oxidative killing of bacteria. The immunoglobulin levels are usually normal.

162   B: Elevated fibrinogen levels

Disseminated intravascular coagulation (DIC) is a syndrome arising as a complication of many different serious and life-threatening illnesses such as septicaemia, as in this case. In its acute (overt) form it is a haemorrhagic disorder, characterised by multiple ecchymoses, mucosal, venepuncture-site and visceral bleeding, and depletion of platelets and clotting factors in the blood. Tissues may become ischaemic. Coagulation abnormalities include: prolonged prothrombin time, activated partial thromboplastin time, thrombin time; decreased fibrinogen levels; increased levels of fibrinogen degradation products (FDP) and d-dimer. The platelet count is decreased as a rule but as it may be falling from a higher level, it may still be normal. Schistocytes will be seen on a peripheral blood smear.

163   B: Graves' disease

Bilateral proptosis is almost certainly due to Graves' disease. The most common cause of a unilateral proptosis is also Graves' disease but, not uncommonly, other diseases may be responsible. Although Graves' disease is linked to thyroid problems, it is possible to be hyperthyroid, hypothyroid or euthyroid and still have Graves'-related eye disease. Other causes of proptosis include cavernous hemangioma, lymphangioma, lymphoma, Wegener's granulomatosis, histiocytosis X, optic nerve glioma, orbital cellulitis and orbital pseudotumour.

164   E: Spirometry

Recognition of COPD in its early stages is possible with the use of lung function testing, particularly spirometry. The characteristic findings include reduction in forced expiratory volume in one second (FEV_1), the forced vital capacity (FVC) and the ratio of these two measurements (FEV_1/FVC). The reversibility with bronchodilators test is usually negative.

While peak flow monitoring is recommended in patients with asthma, for many reasons it should not be used in place of spirometry to detect or monitor lung function in COPD. Compared with spirometry, peak flow monitoring is relatively insensitive in detecting early and mild airway obstruction, is more dependent on patient effort (having twice the interpatient and intrapatient variability), and is much less accurate. By the time any abnormalities are seen on the chest X-ray, COPD is in its end stages. High-resolution computed tomographic scanning is not cost-effective in the early detection of COPD, but several reports suggest that it may be very useful in the early detection of lung cancer, a disease also caused by smoking, which often coexists with COPD. The electrocardiogram is not useful in early detection of COPD because abnormalities are usually present only in the late stages.

165 E: Treatment with penicillin should be initiated without delay

Brucellosis, a bacterial zoonosis, is a disease that is caused by the bacterial genus *Brucella*. Ingestion of unpasteurised goat's milk and related dairy products is the main route of *B. melitensis* transmission to humans. The most common findings are hepatosplenomegaly (or isolated hepatomegaly or splenomegaly) and osteoarticular involvement. Spondylitis of the sacroiliac joint and discitis of the spine are not uncommon features of the disease. Standard culturing techniques require prolonged incubation periods under special conditions; so, if clinically suspected, notify laboratory personnel of your concern about brucellosis so that proper specimen processing is expedited.

The use of doxycycline and rifampicin for four to six weeks is the therapy of choice. *Brucella* species are small, slow-growing, coccobacillary Gram-negative intracellular aerobes. Treatment with penicillin is not effective.

166 C: Festinant gait

The neck spasm is most likely to be an acute dystonic reaction to antipsychotic medication. All antipsychotic medications are associated with the development of Parkinsonian features: this is most marked with drugs such as haloperidol and trifluoperazine and least marked with the newer 'atypicals' such as clozapine. Festinant gait, resting tremor and cogwheel rigidity are the cardinal features.

167 B: A reduction in heart size

Dobutamine and dopamine are non-digitalis positive inotropic drugs currently approved for short-term use in congestive heart failure. The most obvious deleterious effect of a failing heart is the inability to pump enough blood to satisfy the energy requirements of all the body tissues. Among the compensatory mechanisms that develop in response to heart failure is an increase in retention of fluid by the kidney. Increased retention of fluid causes the end diastolic volume to increase which, by the Starling mechanism, increases the strength of the heartbeat. However, two deleterious effects result from an increase in end-diastolic volume. A larger than normal end-diastolic volume causes an increase in end-diastolic pressure which can lead to pulmonary oedema. In addition the large end-diastolic volume increases the wall stress that must be developed by the heart with each beat, and this increases the myocardial requirement for oxygen. The increase in contractility produced by positive inotropic drugs allows the heart to produce the same force at a lower volume, and thus eliminate the need for an increase in volume of fluid.

168 D: Plasma cell invasion of the kidney

Renal disease is a common problem in multiple myeloma, although a variety of different mechanisms may be involved. There is also a general correlation between the presence and severity of renal disease and patient survival. Amyloid light chain amyloidosis can occur in the kidney and can cause nephrotic syndrome. Renal disease can also arise from the formation in the tubules of casts which contain immunoglobulin light chains. Hypercalcaemia can contribute to the development of renal failure by causing renal vasoconstriction, by leading to intratubular calcium deposition, and perhaps by increasing the toxicity of filtered light chains. Renal failure is a potential, although infrequent, complication of radiocontrast administration in patients with multiple myeloma. Prior volume depletion and urinary light chain excretion are present in almost all cases: the former may predispose to contrast nephropathy by enhancing light chain precipitation within the tubules. Plasma cell invasion of the kidney can occur in multiple myeloma, but it is rarely severe enough to impair renal function.

169 E: Loss of the ankle jerk

The common peroneal nerve is a branch of the sciatic nerve. It winds around the neck of the fibula before dividing into the superficial and deep peroneal nerves. The latter is responsible for eversion of the ankle and dorsiflexion of the foot (patient can't walk on their heel). Inversion is not lost as this is partially controlled by the tibialis posterior supplied by the tibial nerve. Sensation to the sole of the foot is supplied by the medial and lateral plantar branches of the tibial nerve. Loss of the ankle jerk is a feature of injury to the sciatic nerve or its tibial branch.

170 A: Lymphocyte

Plasma cells are differentiated cells of B lymphocyte cell lineage. Most plasma cells are thought to complete their differentiation in the bone marrow. Plasma cells in the bone marrow are derived from germinal centre B cells, which are destined to be either memory B cells or plasma cells. Plasma cells are regarded as a type of lymphocyte that produces the immunoglobulin (antibody) that is necessary for normal immune system function.

171 C: Catalase

Some bacteria and macrophages can reduce diatomic oxygen to hydrogen peroxide or superoxide. Both of these molecules are toxic to bacteria. Some bacteria, however, possess a defence mechanism which can minimise the harm done by the two compounds. These resistant bacteria use two enzymes to catalyse the conversion of hydrogen peroxide and superoxide back into diatomic oxygen and water. One of these enzymes is catalase and its presence can be detected by a simple test. The catalase test involves adding hydrogen peroxide to a culture sample or agar slant. If the bacteria in question produce catalase, they will convert the hydrogen peroxide and oxygen gas will be formed. The evolution of gas causes bubbles to form and is indicative of a positive test. Catalase is found in most aerobic and facultative anaerobic bacteria. The main exceptions are *Streptococcus* spp. Catalase is not found in anaerobes.

The coagulase test is a method for differentiating between pathogenic and non-pathogenic strains of *Staphylococcus*. Urease is an enzyme that breaks the carbon–nitrogen bond of amides to form carbon dioxide, ammonia and water. *Proteus* species are known to produce urease. The indole test is used in the differentiation of genera and species, for example to differentiate *Escherichia coli* (+) from enterobacteria (–) or *Proteus mirabilis* (–) from other *Proteus* species. The oxidase test is useful in the differentiation of enterobacteria (–) and *Pseudomonas* (+). Remember that an oxidase-positive organism will be catalase-positive.

172 B: A decrease in calcium

Parathyroid hormone is released in response to low extracellular concentrations of free calcium. Changes in blood phosphate concentration can be associated with changes in parathyroid hormone secretion, but this appears to be an indirect effect and phosphate *per se* is not a significant regulator of this hormone.

173 B: Mast cells

Anaphylaxis refers to a severe allergic reaction in which prominent dermal and systemic signs and symptoms are manifest. The full-blown syndrome includes urticaria (hives) and/or angio-oedema, with hypotension and bronchospasm. Food is the most common cause of anaphylaxis, but insect stings, medicine, latex or exercise can also cause a reaction. In the classic form, mediator release (histamine, leukotriene C4, prostaglandin D2 and tryptase) occurs when the antigen (allergen) binds to antigen-specific immunoglobulin E (IgE) attached to previously sensitised basophils and mast cells. In an anaphylactoid reaction, exposure to an inciting substance causes direct release of mediators, a process that is not mediated by IgE.

174 C: Osteomalacia

Osteomalacia is caused by insufficient levels of vitamin D in the body. It usually presents with widespread bone pains and sometimes muscle weakness. Fractures can occur. Inadequate exposure to sunlight and low dietary intake are usually necessary for the development of clinical vitamin D deficiency. Elderly people who are housebound or confined to residential and nursing homes are particularly susceptible. Osteomalacia must be differentiated from other causes of widespread bone decalcification (eg hyperparathyroidism, senile or postmenopausal osteoporosis, Cushing's syndrome, multiple myeloma or atrophy of disuse). Low 25-hydroxyvitamin D_3 levels, low serum calcium and phosphate, raised alkaline phosphatase and parathyroid hormone, together with X-ray findings of demineralisation (pseudofractures, Looser's lines, Milkman's syndrome) confirm the diagnosis.

Although the patient's back pain could be explained by any of the suggested diagnoses, osteoporosis is not usually accompanied by calcium abnormalities. Multiple myeloma and primary hyperparathyroidism more frequently present with hypercalcaemia; renal failure should have manifested other signs, apart from the hypocalcaemia.

175 D: High serum lipid levels

Creatinine is a breakdown product of creatine, which is an important constituent of muscle. Creatinine is released into the blood. The amount produced is relatively stable in a given person. The creatinine level in the serum is therefore determined by the rate at which it is being removed, which is roughly a measure of kidney function. If kidney function falls (say, a kidney is removed to donate to a relative), the creatinine level will rise. However, other factors affect the serum creatinine levels. Serum creatinine levels are increased by: renal insufficiency; decreased renal perfusion; urinary tract infections; skeletal muscle trauma or rhabdomyolysis; diabetic ketoacidosis and drugs (inhibit tubular secretion of creatinine), eg aminoglycosides, cephalosporin, cefoxitin, cephalothin, hydantoin, diuretics, methyldopa, cimetidine and trimethoprim. Serum creatinine levels are decreased by decreased muscle mass (late-stage muscular dystrophy) and in pregnancy.

176 C: Varicella antibody testing should be performed because it is likely that he is already immune

About 80% of adults who recall no history of chickenpox are immune due to forgotten or subclinical illness. Adults should therefore be tested for varicella immunity before proceeding with immunisation when there is no history of chickenpox. Vaccination is reasonable in men younger than 30 years who are motivated to comply with testing followed by vaccination if they are antibody-negative. Adults with chickenpox frequently have severe symptoms and are at greater risk of developing complications compared with children.

177 A: Potassium levels

This patient is quite young to be presenting with osteoporosis and he should be evaluated for secondary causes of this problem. Basic tests should include a full blood count, kidney and liver function tests, vitamin D and calcium level measurements, measurements of sex hormones, protein electrophoresis and thyroid hormone levels. Electrolytic abnormalities (of sodium, potassium or magnesium) have not been associated with osteoporosis.

178 D: Calcium gluconate, intravenously

The acute treatment utilises agents that either stabilise cardiac cells in the face of hyperkalaemia or shift potassium intracellularly, to acutely lower extracellular (ie plasma) levels. The most appropriate initial therapy entails the stabilisation of excitable cardiac membranes with calcium gluconate, administered intravenously. This intervention often reverses the abnormal changes on the electrocardiogram. However, this effect is short-lived (approximately 30 minutes), and the treatment may need to be repeated.

A reduction in serum potassium is the next step in the treatment. Bicarbonate causes hydrogen ions to leave cells to maintain the proper plasma pH, which in turn prompts potassium entry into cells in order to maintain electroneutrality. This effect is typically seen after 30 to 60 minutes. Intravenous administration of insulin plus glucose is the most effective therapy for lowering serum potassium, by shifting this cation into cells. Removal of excess potassium from the body can also be achieved through the gastrointestinal tract with sodium polystyrene sulfonate resin, which exchanges Ca^{++} in the resin for K^+ from the body or through the blood by haemodialysis and these might be used in conjunction with the above measures. Loop or thiazide diuretics enhance renal excretion of potassium, though this may be of limited use in patients in whom renal failure was the cause of hyperkalaemia in the first place.

179 B: Low birth weight

Fetal alcohol syndrome is a lifelong yet completely preventable set of physical, mental and neurobehavioural birth defects associated with maternal alcohol consumption during pregnancy. The diagnosis of fetal alcohol syndrome can only be made when the patient shows signs of abnormality in each of the three categories: prenatal and/or postnatal growth retardation (weight and/or length below the 10th percentile when corrected for gestational age); central nervous system involvement, including neurological abnormality, developmental delay, behavioural dysfunction or deficit, intellectual impairment and/or structural abnormalities, such as microcephaly (head circumference below the 3rd percentile) or brain malformations found on imaging studies or autopsy; and a characteristic face, with short palpebral fissures, an elongated mid-face, a long and flattened philtrum, thin upper lip, and a flattened maxilla.

180 B: Ankle clonus

The cauda equina is a collection of intradural nerve roots beginning at the end of the spinal cord. *Cauda* is Latin for 'tail', and *equina* is Latin for 'horse', ie the 'horse's tail'. A positive Babinski sign, ankle clonus or other signs of upper motor neurone involvement suggest a diagnosis other than cauda equine syndrome, possibly spinal cord compression. Poor anal sphincter tone is characteristic of the syndrome. Muscle weakness may be present in muscles supplied by affected roots. Pain is often localised to the low back; local tenderness on palpation or percussion may be present. Reflex abnormalities may be present, typically including loss or diminution of reflexes.

A typical history includes the following features:

- low back pain, usually in the form of common symptoms of bilateral sciatica
- unilateral or bilateral lower extremity motor and/or sensory abnormality
- bowel and/or bladder dysfunction
- a difference in feeling when wiping after a bowel movement, usually associated with saddle (perineal) anaesthesia.

181 D: Hypercitraturia

Increased citrate is a protective factor against calcium stones. An increased intake of citrate is recommended for prophylaxis in many patients with calcium stones. Most kidney stones are calcium oxalate stones. Calcium oxalate urinary stones may be associated with any one of several causes of hypercalcaemia, which could also lead to hypercalciuria. Some patients with calcium stones may have associated hyperuricosuria as a cause of their stone. Some 10–20% of patients with gout may have kidney stones containing uric acid, calcium oxalate or phosphate, or a combination. Hypercalciuria is the cause of at least 50% of all kidney stones. Patients with calcium oxalate stones and normal urinary calcium should be investigated for hyperuricaemia.

182 C: 200 mg/day

Microalbuminuria is defined as the excretion of > 30 mg albumin/day but < 300 mg albumin/day. Urinary protein consists of albumin, low-molecular-weight proteins filtered from blood and urinary tract-derived proteins. Proteinuria in glomerular diseases is mostly due to increased albumin excretion. It is preferable to measure albuminuria rather than proteinuria for chronic kidney disease in adults. The normal mean value for albumin excretion for healthy adults is 10 mg/day. However, the upper limit of normal is arbitrarily set at 30 mg/day.

183 E: Eosinophils in the urine

Although eosinophils in the urine may be seen in patients with glomerulonephritis, this finding is not specific and they may be seen in patients with interstitial nephritis and prostatitis. Dysmorphic RBCs and RBC casts suggest a glomerular source and urological evaluation is not needed in these patients. Heavy proteinuria with haematuria is also suggestive of glomerular disease. Lipiduria is a feature of nephrotic syndrome.

184 A: Haematuria

The classic presentation of nephrotic syndrome is a low serum albumin (it is lost in the urine), a high serum cholesterol and over 3 g of proteinuria per 24 hours. Oval fat bodies may be seen in the urine. A finding of blood in the urine is not necessary to diagnose nephrotic syndrome.

185 B: Light chain immunoglobulins in the urine
Most of the routine dipstick methods for measuring albumin and protein do not detect other urinary proteins as well as they detect albumin. Light chains are not usually detected by urine dipstick methods. Urine that is highly alkaline may react with the dipstick to cause a false-positive reaction. Radiocontrast material will cause a false-positive test on dipstick and by sulphosalicylic acid. Each of the other choices may cause an increase in urinary albumin/protein.

186 B: Vitamin B$_{12}$
Short bowel syndrome occurs after an extensive resection of the small bowel. Patients with this problem present with chronic diarrhoea, dehydration, electrolyte abnormalities and malnutrition as a result of severe maldigestion and malabsorption. The most common causes of short bowel syndrome in adults are Crohn's disease, mesenteric ischaemia and complications of cancer therapy. The bulk of nutrient absorption takes place in the first 150 cm of the small bowel in the region of the duodenum and proximal jejunum. The length of the small bowel in adults ranges from 365 to 600 cm. When the extent of intestinal resection is considered, less than 50% can be tolerated quite well; 50% to 75% often requires dietary manipulation, oral supplementation and medications to enhance intestinal absorption; and greater than 75% often requires prolonged parenteral nutrition. The duodenum is the site where calcium, magnesium, iron and folate are preferentially absorbed. The distal 100 cm of the ileum is the only region of the small bowel where vitamin B$_{12}$–intrinsic factor complex is absorbed. This patient would not be expected to be deficient in B$_{12}$.

187 E: Chest X-ray
This patient is presenting with chest infection and physical signs of consolidation. Pneumonia is the most likely diagnosis but a similar presentation could be due to bronchial carcinoma or pulmonary tuberculosis. A full blood count might show a raised white cell count, but this abnormality is non-specific and may occur in bronchial carcinoma and tuberculosis. The physical signs are not typical of pleural effusion and thoracentesis should not be attempted without a radiological confirmation of pleural effusion. Chest X-rays would not only help to verify the clinical finding of consolidation but also might give a clue to the possible underlying pathology, for example rib destruction and lymphadenopathy in bronchial carcinoma or cavity formation and nodular shadows in tuberculosis. HIV testing has no role in the initial stages of

assessment but would be very helpful in further specification of the specific type of infection (eg *Pneumocystis carinii* pneumonia). Liver tests are abnormal in most cases of pneumonia as well as in malignancy with metastasis and in tuberculosis, so they are non-specific.

188 **D: Withhold warfarin therapy and administer vitamin K₁ 3 mg orally**

In this case the patient's INR elevation was possibly due to antibiotic therapy, either due to pharmacokinetic effects or to suppression of the intestinal flora that produce vitamin K. The recommendation with an INR > 9.0 with no significant bleeding is to withhold warfarin therapy and administer vitamin K_1 3–5 mg orally, with the expectation that the INR will be reduced substantially in 24–48 hours. Monitor the INR every 24 hours and administer additional vitamin K_1 if necessary. Resume therapy at a lower dose when the INR reaches the therapeutic range.

189 **A: Coeliac sprue**

Uraemia and primary biliary cirrhosis are serious considerations in someone with chronic itching. Dry skin caused by dry weather may seem like an obvious potential cause of her itching, but in this case is less likely because her symptoms have been present for several months. Oral contraceptives have been associated with itching in certain parts of the world (Scandinavia and Chile). Coeliac sprue is not associated with itching but with a skin disorder, dermatitis herpetiformis, which usually presents as itchy vesicular lesions with intense burning.

190 **D: Begin low molecular weight heparin subcutaneously; begin warfarin on day three**

Heparin should be started immediately. Low molecular weight heparin is as effective as unfractionated heparin and may be less costly, allowing the patient to be cared for at home. Although many may recommend starting heparin and warfarin together, the rare complication of thrombosis may occur in the patient with protein C deficiency. This can usually be obviated if warfarin is started after day two.

Aspirin is used for proplylaxis in patients at high risk for deep venous thrombosis (DVT). It should be taken before setting off on a long flight. Thrombolytic therapy is preserved for more severe proximal DVTs and for massive pulmonary embolism. Unfortunately, there is a 1–2% risk of developing an intracranial bleed with thrombolysis of venous thromboembolism.

It has been shown that there is a direct relationship between distance travelled in a passenger aircraft and the risk for pulmonary embolism. For those traveling < 5000 km (< 3100 miles) the risk is 0.01 case/million passengers; > 5000 km this risk is 1.5/million; and > 10, 000 km the risk is 4.8 cases/million.

191 E: Postmenopausal women
The risk of osteoporosis increases at the menopause and Caucasian women are at the greatest risk. Osteoporosis will affect one in three women after the age of 50 but screening all postmenopausal women is not cost-effective. They need not have screening unless there are other associated risk factors. Patients taking more than 5 mg prednisolone for more than 12 weeks should be screened as should those with primary biliary cirrhosis (usually women), those with hypogonadism, and those with osteoporosis-associated fractures.

192 C: The presence of secondary gain
Munchausen's syndrome is a factitious disorder. This disorder is defined as the voluntary production of physical or psychological symptoms, which can be attributed to a need to adopt the sick role. Secondary gain is defined as the presence of an advantage gained as a result of having symptoms – in this case, attention and admission. Munchausen's syndrome differs from malingering in that there is no fraudulent simulation of symptoms. Financial gain is therefore not a motive. Alcohol dependence may be present but is not particularly associated with the syndrome. This condition should not be confused with hypochondria, in which the person visits many doctors in the belief that he or she is sick. In Munchausen's syndrome the individual knows that the illness does not exist but chooses to gain attention that cannot be realised in any other way.

193 D: Female gender
The natural history of hepatitis C virus (HCV) infection varies from person to person. Generally, chronic infection will develop in about 60%–85% of patients with the disease. Factors associated with spontaneous clearance of infection include young age at the time of infection and female gender. Accelerated progression to chronic liver disease is associated with male sex, older age at time of infection, alcohol intake, and co-infection with other viruses, including HIV. Viral genotypes 2 and 3 are associated with a better response in virus load to antiviral therapy.

194 C: Bernard–Soulier syndrome

The bleeding time is a measure of the interaction of platelets with the blood vessel wall. A prolonged bleeding time is seen in thrombocytopenia (platelet count is usually below $50 \times 10^9/l$) or qualitative platelet abnormalities. Among patients with a normal platelet count, measuring the bleeding time is recommended primarily to screen patients for inherited disorders of platelet function. An abnormal test in a patient with mucocutaneous bleeding would justify further testing for platelet dysfunction or specific tests for von Willebrand's disease. Bernard–Soulier syndrome is a hereditary intrinsic platelet disorder. It is an autosomal recessive disorder that affects surface membrane glycoproteins. Unusually large platelets are present that do not agglutinate with ristocetin but aggregate normally with the physiological aggregating agents ADP, collagen and adrenaline (epinephrine). Large platelets are associated with functional abnormalities and a prolonged bleeding time.

195 C: Dual-energy X-ray absorptiometry (DEXA) bone density measurement

Certain findings in patients with primary hyperparathyroidism influence the physician's decision on whether or not to perform surgery. Apart from the symptomatic patient, especially one in hypercalcaemic crisis, other indications for surgery include kidney stones, osteoporosis, renal impairment, and young age. To determine the first three of these factors, general biochemical tests, ultrasonography of the kidneys and DEXA bone density measurements are usually performed. Localisation of the parathyroid adenoma is considered only when surgery is contemplated.

196 D: Unwilling to monitor his own blood glucose levels

The goals of intensive therapy can be achieved either by multiple daily injections (MDI) of insulin or by continuous subcutaneous insulin infusion (CSII) by means of an insulin pump. The disadvantages of MDI are that three or more injections are needed daily and intermediate and long-acting insulins (NPH, lente, ultralente, or glargine) must be used as the basal component. Absorption of the modified insulins has been shown to vary from 19% to 55% in the same individual, resulting in variable glucose levels. In contrast, absorption of the soluble, short-acting insulins that are used in CSII varies by less than 3% daily.

Pump therapy is now regarded as a safe and viable alternative in adults, adolescents and children with diabetes. The main advantage of CSII over MDI is better insulin pharmacokinetics. With CSII, only short-acting insulin is used, all food intake (primarily carbohydrates) is covered by insulin boluses given by the user, and normal blood glucose levels are maintained at other times by continuous delivery of basal insulin. Other advantages of CSII include decreased variability in insulin absorption; decreased risk of nocturnal hypoglycaemia and improved control of the dawn phenomenon with use of variable basal rates; greater freedom in timing of meals and snacks and decreased risk of activity-induced hypoglycaemia. CSII therefore simulates the function of the islet cells more closely than MDI. However, the most important factor for successful treatment with insulin pumps is the frequency of blood glucose monitoring. Patients who monitor blood glucose levels three or more times a day have a lower average Hb A_{1c} level than patients who monitor levels once or twice daily. Therefore, diabetics who have difficulties with frequent monitoring of their blood glucose levels would not gain any added benefit from pump therapy and should not be prescribed this form of intensive therapy. In brief, the indications for insulin pump therapy include:

- A history of hypoglycaemic unawareness or hypoglycaemic events requiring assistance
- Need for flexibility in lifestyle (eg shift workers, business travellers, workers in a safety-sensitive job)
- Pregnancy (or planned pregnancy).

197 B: PR interval

The vagal fibres innervating the heart stimulate intracardiac postganglionic fibres, which release acetylcholine. The postganglionic fibres innervate the sinoatrial and atrioventricular (AV) nodal fibres. Acetycholine causes a decrease in the rate of phase 4 depolarisation, thus slowing the heart, and a decrease in conduction velocity through the AV node, thus increasing the PR interval. Acetycholine also causes a slight decrease in contractility. Decreasing the heart rate increases the amount of time available for ventricle filling and thus increases the end-diastolic volume. However, the end-systolic volume will be somewhat elevated because of the slight decrease in contractility and increase in afterload. The ejection fraction will therefore remain the same or decrease slightly.

198   E: Schizophrenia

Prodromal schizophrenia often includes social withdrawal and behaviour change. The initial presentation, before the onset of delusions and hallucinations, may be subtle. The presence of odd ideas, as in this case the belief that his mother is trying to poison him, needs to be explored in order to confirm whether they are delusional. Delusions are beliefs that are held with absolute certainty. They are usually false and not understandable in the context of a person's cultural and social background. Delusions can occur in severe depression, and amphetamine use. Depressive delusions are usually congruent with the mood and have themes of guilt or hopelessness.

199   A: Secretion of large amounts of chloride in the small intestine

Cholera (frequently called 'Asiatic cholera' or 'epidemic cholera') is a severe diarrhoeal disease caused by the bacterium *Vibrio cholerae*. Transmission to humans is by water or food. *V. cholerae* produces cholera toxin, the model for enterotoxins, whose action on the mucosal epithelium is responsible for the characteristic diarrhoea of the disease cholera. The net effect of the toxin is to cause cAMP to be produced at an abnormally high rate which stimulates mucosal cells to pump large amounts of chloride into the intestinal contents. Water, sodium and other electrolytes follow due to the osmotic and electrical gradients caused by the loss of chloride. The lost water and electrolytes in mucosal cells are replaced from the blood. The toxin-damaged cells therefore become pumps for water and electrolytes, causing the diarrhoea, loss of electrolytes and dehydration that are characteristic of cholera.

200   E: Temporal lobe

The hippocampus is part of the limbic system, which is formed from the medial parts of the temporal, parietal and frontal lobes. The hippocampus is intimately associated with memory and lesions within this area of the brain will lead to a variety of memory disorders, including amnesia.

PAPER THREE ANSWERS

201 A: Smallpox virus

The Herpesvirus family includes:

- Herpes simplex type I (HSV-1)
- Herpes simplex type II (HSV-2)
- Varicella zoster virus (VZV)
- Human cytomegalovirus (CMV)
- Epstein–Barr virus (EBV)
- Human herpesvirus 6 (HHV6)
- Human herpesvirus 7 (HHV7)
- Human herpesvirus 8 (HHV8)

The smallpox virus is a linear double-stranded DNA from the Poxviridae family.

202 D: Actinic keratosis is more common in fair-skinned individuals

Exposure to UV radiation is a major cause of actinic keratoses, which are among the strongest determinants of skin cancer risk. Most people with fair skin, especially those who sunburn easily and tan poorly and those whose occupations or hobbies result in excessive sun exposure are at increased risk of developing actinic keratoses, which might develop into squamous cell carcinoma. Physicians should be prepared to advise patients about cutaneous photoprotection, the major way to prevent the development of skin cancers. These protective measures include remaining indoors; exposing the skin to sunlight only at times when UV radiation is relatively weak; wearing clothing protective against UV radiation penetration; using topical sunscreens; and taking or applying medications. To avoid sunlight whenever it is likely to produce unwanted effects usually means minimising sun exposure between 10 or 11 am and 3 or 4 pm, even on cloudy or cool days. Commercial sunscreens cause little contact dermatitis, no systemic problems through absorption, and no secondary vitamin D deficiency. SLE has no single known cause. People with SLE are often photosensitive and they could develop rash, fever, joint pain or other symptoms. However, sun exposure is often linked to flare-up of established SLE and not as a definite cause of the disease.

203   D: Its endogenous levels are dramatically reduced on exposure to intense artificial light

Melatonin is a naturally occurring hormone released by the pineal gland. Melatonin levels respond to an individual's natural circadian rhythms by increasing late in the afternoon/early evening and decreasing dramatically during the day. Light exposure, either natural or artificial, causes extremely rapid destruction of the hormone. It has long been assumed that melatonin is responsible for sleep regulation, though the exact mechanism of action remains unknown. Melatonin is able to help shift your body clock to earlier or later times. For example, when travelling eastwards you need to sleep, eat and work earlier than in your home time zone and when traveling westwards you need to sleep, eat and work later. It also reinforces the effects of darkness by increasing sleepiness, decreasing alertness and lowering your temperature slightly. It is not a sedative but has hypnotic properties. Melatonin can induce sleep at the correct time and is used in individuals with jet lag syndrome, and for insomnia in blind or elderly people and shift workers.

Melatonin can cause alteration in melanin pigment distribution in animals. Although such cutaneous effects of melatonin are seen in a variety of 'lower species', the hormone does not have such effects in mammals or birds. Melatonin might have anti-ageing effects. Levels of melatonin are, on average, double in young people than what they are in people in their fifties. It is an antioxidant, like vitamins C and E, which neutralise dangerous molecules known as free radicals, which might be responsible for the ageing process.

204   D: Inhibits factor Xa

Patients with a diagnosis of acute deep venous thrombosis have traditionally been hospitalised and treated with unfractionated heparin followed by oral anticoagulation therapy. Several clinical trials have shown that low molecular weight heparin (LMWH) is at least as safe and effective as unfractionated heparin in the treatment of uncomplicated deep venous thrombosis. The use of LMWHs in an outpatient programme for the management of deep venous thrombosis provides a treatment alternative to hospitalisation in selected patients.

LMWHs are derived from depolymerisation of standard heparin, which yields fragments approximately one-third of the size of the parent compound. These lower molecular weight fractions have several properties that differentiate them from unfractionated heparin. LMWHs exert their anticoagulant effect by inhibiting factor

Xa and augmenting tissue-factor-pathway inhibitor but minimally affect thrombin, or factor IIa. The APTT, a measure of antithrombin (anti-factor IIa) activity, is therefore not used to measure the activity of LMWHs, which requires instead a specific anti-Xa assay.

205 A: Hay fever

Outside factors, including weather, stress, injury and infection, while not direct causes, are often important in triggering the disease process leading to the onset or worsening of psoriasis.

The weather is a strong factor in psoriasis: cold, dry weather is a common precipitant of psoriasis flares; hot, damp, sunny weather helps relieve the problem in most patients. To confuse matters, however, some people have photosensitive psoriasis, which actually improves in winter and worsens in summer, when skin is exposed to sunlight.

Stress, unexpressed anger and emotional disorders, including depression and anxiety, are strongly associated with psoriasis flares. In one study, nearly 40% of patients remembered a specific stressful event that occurred within a month of a psoriasis flare. Some studies have suggested that patients with psoriasis respond to stress differently from people without the skin disease. In one study, psoriasis patients had fewer aggressive verbal responses than others when confronted with circumstances designed to provoke anger.

Infections caused by viruses or bacteria can trigger some cases of psoriasis. For example streptococcal infections in the upper respiratory tract, such as tonsillitis, sinusitis and so-called 'strep' throat, are known to trigger psoriasis, particularly guttate psoriasis, in people with a specific genetic type (HLA-B13). The human immunodeficiency virus (HIV) is also associated with psoriasis.

Although experts have sought a bacterial or viral agent as a cause of pustular psoriasis, none have been identified so far.

The Koebner response is a delayed response at the site of previous injuries (eg cuts, burns, injections, previous skin disorders), in which psoriasis then develops. In some cases, even mild abrasions can cause an eruption, which may be a factor in the high frequency of psoriasis on the elbows or knees. (It should be noted that psoriasis can develop in areas with no history of skin disruption.)

A number of drugs can worsen or induce pre-existing latent psoriasis, including the anti-malarial drug chloroquine; certain drugs used for hypertension and heart problems, including angiotensin-converting enzyme (ACE) inhibitors and β-blockers, which may actually trigger the onset of psoriasis and produce flares in people who already have it; progesterone; lithium, which is used in bipolar disorder, and may trigger the onset of the disease and cause severe flares in people who already have psoriasis; and indometacin, a non-steroidal anti-inflammatory drug (NSAID) (although other NSAIDs, such as meclofenamate, may actually improve the condition). Withdrawing from oral steroids or high-potency steroid ointments that cover wide skin areas can cause flare-ups of severe psoriasis, including guttate, pustular and erythrodermic psoriasis. Because these drugs are also used to treat psoriasis, this rebound effect is of particular concern. Drugs that cause rashes can also trigger psoriasis as part of the Koebner response.

Hay fever is not usually associated with psoriasis flares.

206 B: Blood glucose levels

Iritis can occur at any age. In children it is most commonly associated with a form of juvenile arthritis. In young adults it can be associated with certain rheumatological disorders, such as ankylosing spondylitis and Reiter's syndrome. 25% of patients with sarcoidosis have eye lesions, iritis being one of the commonest in this disorder. Certain infections, such as tuberculosis, Lyme disease and syphilis, can also cause iritis. However, for most patients, there is no associated underlying condition. In particular, there appears to be no link between diabetes and iritis.

207 C: Toluene diisocyanate

Exposure to general environmental pollution, as well as to specific carcinogenic substances, increases the risk of lung cancer. In particular, several occupational materials are hazardous. These include asbestos, chloromethyl ether, ionising radiation and polycyclic aromatic hydrocarbons. Exposure to radon gas also results in an increased risk of lung cancer. Some of these compounds combine synergistically with tobacco smoke to create a much higher risk. For example, smokers exposed to asbestos have nearly 60 times the risk for lung cancer compared with smokers not exposed to asbestos.

Toluene diisocyanate exposure during production of polyurethane may produce persistent asthma in susceptible individuals.

208 D: Band forms

Malaria occurs in most tropical regions of the world with *Plasmodium falciparum* infection predominating in Africa, New Guinea and Haiti. In *P. vivax*, *P. ovale* and probably *P. malariae* infections, all stages of development subsequent to the liver cycle can be observed in the peripheral blood. However, in the case of

P. falciparum infection, only ring forms and gametocytes are usually present in the peripheral blood. Developing forms appear to stick in the blood vessels of the large organs, such as the brain, and restrict the blood flow with serious consequences. In *P. falciparum* malaria the red cells are not enlarged. Rings appear fine and delicate and there may be several in one cell. Some rings may have two chromatin dots. There may be marginal or applique forms. It is unusual to see developing forms in peripheral blood films. Gametocytes have a characteristic crescent-shape appearance. However, they do not usually appear in the blood for the first four weeks of infection. Maurer's dots may be present. Band forms are a characteristic of *P. malariae* infection Ring forms may have a squarish appearance.

209 A: Parvovirus B19 infection

An adult who is not immune and comes in contact with a child who has a viral infection such as parvovirus B19 (slapped cheeks syndrome) can be infected with parvovirus B19 and either have no symptoms or develop the typical rash of fifth disease, or joint pain or swelling (or both). Usually, joints on both sides of the body are affected. The joints most frequently affected are the hands, wrists and knees. The joint pain and swelling usually resolve in a week or two, but they may last several months. If IgM antibody to parvovirus B19 is detected, the test result suggests that the person has had a recent infection. The other diseases mentioned are valid but remote alternative diagnoses and the patient should therefore be reassured that her illness is self-limiting and will cause no long-term damage to her joints.

210 A: Blocking conduction through the atrioventricular (AV) node

Adenosine is an endogenous nucleoside primarily formed as a degradation product of adenosine triphosphate (ATP). As an intermediate metabolite in several biochemical pathways, adenosine contributes to the regulation of numerous physiological processes, including platelet function, coronary and systemic vascular tone, and lipolysis in adipocytes. Early studies in animals demonstrated that adenosine produced a transient slowing of the sinus rate and atrioventricular (AV) block. Subsequently, numerous studies have confirmed the transient negative dromotropic and chronotropic effects of adenosine in both animals and humans. The effect appeared to be mediated by depression of calcium-mediated slow-channel conduction, an increase in potassium conduction, and possibly by an indirect anti-adrenergic effect. Transient AV block is produced by breaking the re-entry circuit within the AV node. Adenosine has no effect on anterograde conduction over accessory pathways in patients with Wolff–Parkinson–White syndrome.

211   C: Involvement of the descending aorta

Dissection of the thoracic aorta is an uncommon but potentially catastrophic event which requires early diagnosis and prompt treatment if the patient is to survive and escape complications (during the early hours of dissection, the hourly mortality rate is more than 1%). The dissection begins as a tear of the intima, most commonly in the ascending aorta and is followed by the creation of a false lumen in the medial layer of the aortic wall. The consequences include rupture (most commonly into the pericardium, into the left pleural space or into the mediastinum), haematoma formation, or re-entry. The latter is more common in the case of dissection of the descending thoracic aorta. Complications include sudden death (often at home) from haemopericardium, stroke or heart attack, due to involvement of the innominate, left common carotid and coronary arteries respectively. By contrast, when the descending aorta is affected the renal arteries may be involved, causing renal failure. All patients with an acute dissection of the ascending aorta should be considered for surgical treatment. Extensive, irreversible injury to the central nervous system is arguably the only contraindication. The ascending aorta is repaired using a Dacron graft and it is usually possible to repair the aortic valve. If the dissection extends beyond the ascending aorta, the distal anastomosis can be secured during a period of circulatory arrest. If the aortic valve is not normal, it is replaced. The approach to patients with intramural haematoma is similar to that for patients with acute aortic dissection but if the aortic arch is involved in the acute dissection, this too can be resected.

For patients with a dissection of the descending aorta, medical treatment is the initial procedure of choice. This consists of careful monitoring of blood pressure and urinary output in an Intensive Care Unit. Blood pressure is controlled with a continuous infusion of labetalol which has both α- and β-antagonist properties and decreases the rate of ejection from the left ventricle. Surgery is indicated in patients with signs of impending rupture and in those with ischaemia of the legs or abdominal viscera, renal failure, paraperesis or paraplegia. With current techniques, elective resection of the thoracic aorta can be accomplished with an operative mortality of 10–12% and rates of spinal ischaemic injury and renal failure of 3–15%.

212 A: It is safe in benign intracranial hypertension

With the advent of sophisticated imaging techniques, particularly computed tomography (CT) and magnetic resonance imaging (MRI), lumbar puncture (LP) is no longer an important test in the diagnosis of most intracranial mass lesions. This is especially true in view of the potential risk of brain herniation if the intracranial pressure is increased markedly. An LP remains a critical procedure in the diagnosis of CNS infections, subarachnoid haemorrhage and inflammatory diseases. The LP itself can be therapeutic, particularly in benign intracranial hypertension (ie pseudotumour cerebri), in which serial LPs may be used for treatment.

213 B: A nephew has been diagnosed with schizophrenia

There are several well-documented risk factors for schizophrenia. The most important risk factor is genetic, with increased risk associated with an affected first- or second-degree relative. A history of obstetric complications is more common in schizophrenia. A number of migrant groups show an increase in incidence of schizophrenia, relative both to the population left behind and to the population they join. People who develop schizophrenia are more likely to have a history of developmental delay and behavioural and interpersonal difficulties in childhood. There is an equal gender incidence of schizophrenia, although males often present earlier. While most researchers do not believe that substance abuse causes schizophrenia, people who have schizophrenia often abuse alcohol and/or drugs.

214 D: Bacterial biotransformation into virus

As long as antimicrobial drugs are used, drug resistance will remain a challenge. The bacteria is attempting to preserve its species, so, by resisting an antibiotic, it guarantees survival. Antibiotic resistance can be categorised into three types. Firstly, organisms may show natural or intrinsic resistance, resulting in inaccessibility of the drug's target (eg impermeability resistance due to the absence of an adequate transporter, such as aminoglycoside resistance in strict anaerobes. Secondly, mutational resistance may develop, with target-site modification (eg streptomycin resistance caused by mutations in rDNA genes (*rpsL*); β-lactam resistance, caused by a change in PBPs (penicillin-binding proteins)). Thirdly, there is extrachromosomal or acquired resistance (disseminated by plasmids or transposons). This type of resistance may be mediated by target-site modification (see above), reduced permeability or uptake, or by metabolic bypass (eg trimethoprim resistance, caused by overproduction of dihydrofolate reductase or *thi* mutants in *Staphylococcus aureus*).

215 A: The tumour is definitely localised to the adrenals

This is a relatively young patient presenting with severe hypertension. The patient reports periodic episodes that suggest bursts of catecholamine release. In a patient of this age, with this history, a catecholamine-producing tumour (phaeochromocytoma) must be a serious consideration. The patient was treated with α- and β-blockers (catecholamine-receptor blocking agents) for several weeks and had no further paroxysms during that time. In this patient, the elevated adrenaline (epinephrine) in the urine indicated that the tumour was located in the adrenal medulla. Similar tumours may be located outside the adrenal gland. When they are, they are called extra-adrenal paragangliomas rather than phaeochromocytomas, and they produce noradrenaline (norepinephrine) but not adrenaline (epinephrine). Furthermore, phaeochromocytomas may metastasise after a period of time (about 10% do). Early recognition and removal can be curative of the tumour as well as the hypertension.

216 B: Increased cardiac preload

The natriuretic peptides, which include atrial natriuretic peptide (ANP) and brain natriuretic peptide (BNP), help to regulate blood pressure and fluid balance by counterbalancing the renin angiotensin system. While renin and angiotensin raise blood pressure, decrease urine output and cause vasoconstriction, the natriuretic peptides have the opposite effects. Both ANP and BNP increase excretion of sodium and water by increasing glomerular filtration and inhibiting renal sodium resorption. They also decrease secretion of aldosterone and renin and cause vasodilatation, reducing blood pressure and extracellular fluid volume. This will lead to a reduction in cardiac preload and improve cardiac performance.

217 D: Erosions

Lupus arthritis causes pain, stiffness, swelling, tenderness and warmth of joints. Several joints are involved at one time and may include hands, feet, wrists, elbows, knees and ankles. The inflammation is symmetrical in distribution, which means it affects similar joints on both sides of the body. Compared to rheumatoid arthritis, lupus arthritis is less disabling and it usually does not cause severe destruction of the joints. Fewer than 10% of people with lupus arthritis will develop deformities of the hands and feet. These are associated with weakening of cartilage and bone and can be seen in the X-rays of the joints. Referred to as 'Jaccoud-type deformities', these are reversible conditions. X-rays of the joints are usually normal in SLE. Non-specific abnormalities, such as soft tissue swelling and joint space narrowing can often be identified, but the presence of erosions is highly suggestive of rheumatoid arthritis.

218 C: Increase in adipose tissue

Age-related changes in pharmacokinetics often require a change in the dose, frequency and route of administration of antimicrobials, especially for frail elderly people. Despite an age-related decrease in small bowel surface area and an increase in gastric pH, changes in drug absorption tend to be trivial and clinically inconsequential. Plasma albumin concentration decreases slightly with age, although this decrease is usually of little importance. However, disease-related decreases in albumin levels can result in higher concentrations of free drug. Because elderly people have less lean body mass and more body fat than do younger people, water-soluble antimicrobials (eg aminoglycosides, penicillins, cephalosporins, amphotericin B) achieve higher concentrations in plasma and tissue, and fat-soluble antimicrobials (eg chloramphenicol, doxycycline, fluconazole) achieve lower concentrations in the elderly. Biliary excretion of antimicrobials is relatively constant with age.

219 C: *Borrelia burgdorferi*

Varicella-zoster virus is the most commonly associated organism, and increased IgM to herpes simplex has been found in facial nerve palsy. No association was found with CMV, rubella, *Borrelia*, respiratory syncytial virus (RSV), mumps, measles or influenza in one study. However, it is well known that facial nerve palsy (unilateral or bilateral) is associated with Lyme disease and some studies have found increased titres of antibodies to *Borrelia burgdorferi*.

220 B: Lung parenchymal disease and no evidence of lymphadenopathy

If a patient has unilateral hilar lymphadenopathy, mediastinal lympadenopathy with no hilar lymphadenopathy, or presents with lung disease alone and later develops lymphadenopathy, a diagnosis other than sarcoidosis is a strong possibility. In sarcoidosis, there is abnormal lung parenchyma with no lymphadenopathy in 20% of cases. Permanent lung fibrosis is also encountered in 15% of cases.

221 B: The S1, Q3, T3 changes on the 12–lead ECG, when identified, are diagnostic

Autopsy series show that 65–90% of pulmonary emboli arise from the lower extremities. However, the majority of patients with pulmonary embolism have no leg symptoms at the time of diagnosis. Less than 30% of patients have symptoms or signs of lower extremity venous thrombosis. It is recommended that patients with a first thromboembolic event occurring in the setting of reversible or time-limited risk factors (eg immobilisation, surgery, trauma, oestrogen use) should receive warfarin therapy for three to six months. Patients who present with acute massive pulmonary embolism and hypotension have a mortality rate of approximately 20%, despite the use of anticoagulants and other supportive measures. For such patients, the appropriate use of thrombolytic agents has a role. Overall, arterial blood gas measurements do not play a major role in excluding or establishing the diagnosis of pulmonary embolism.

S1, Q3, T3 ECG changes are identified in only 25% of cases. They reflect an increased right ventricular strain due to any cause, and are not specific for pulmonary embolism.

222 C: Increased growth hormone (GH) levels

Anorexia nervosa is associated with a number of physical complications, similar to the effect of starvation. Metabolic and hormonal disturbances can occur. T3 levels may be reduced but TSH and thyroxine levels are usually normal. Gonadotrophin levels are reduced. Growth hormone and plasma cortisol levels are increased, with a loss of the normal diurnal variation of cortisol.

223 B: Order a proteinase 3 (PR3) antibodies ELISA test

The presence of antineutrophil cytoplasmic autoantibodies (ANCA) – antibodies to cytoplasmic proteinase 3 (cANCA) – using indirect immunofluorescence has proven to be highly sensitive for Wegener's granulomatosis. cANCA can be identified in 90% of cases of Wegener's granulomatosis. However, although they are sensitive, their reactions to various enzymes other than proteinase 3 within the cytoplasm render them less specific for Wegener's granulomatosis. Therefore, a more specific test (though less sensitive) has been introduced using the enzyme-linked immunosorbent assay (ELISA) method for detecting anti-proteinase 3 (anti-PR3) antibodies. The ELISA test appears to be more specific for disease diagnosis. Consequently, the current recommendation for testing for Wegener's granulomatosis is the combination of the indirect immunofluorescent test with the antigen-specific ELISA test.

This means a positive indirect immunofluorescent test (cANCA) should be verified with a subsequent anti-PR3 ELISA test.

224 E: Goodpasture's syndrome

Goodpasture's syndrome is uncommon. The patient, most often a young man, characteristically presents with severe haemoptysis, dyspnoea and rapidly progressive renal failure. Chest X-rays may show progressive, bilateral fluffy densities, but rarely demonstrate a cavity in the lung.

225 E: Give no treatment but restart warfarin when INR < 5.0

When the INR is between 6.0 and 8.0 and there is no evidence of bleeding or only minor bleeding as in this patient, the best course of action is to stop warfarin, monitor the INR, and restart warfarin when the INR is less than 5.0.

226 B: 'They control me; they made me take my clothes off'

This is an example of passivity (made) phenomena, one of the 'first rank' symptoms of schizophrenia. In addition to passivity of movement, other made phenomena include passivity of thought and emotions. Other first rank symptoms include some types of auditory hallucinations (in 3rd person, usually talking or arguing about the patient; running commentary; thought echo), thought possession (thought insertion, withdrawal and broadcasting) and delusional perception (attaching a delusional significance to a normal percept). Not all people with schizophrenia have first rank symptoms. 'Transputer' may be an example of a neologism, an invented word strongly suggestive of schizophrenia.

227 A: Inhibiting gyrase enzymes

Quinolones are produced synthetically. They have a nucleus of two fused six-membered rings. Substitutions on this ring characterise the different drugs in this group. They act by blocking the DNA topoisomerases (DNA gyrase is topoisomerase II), enzymes needed for bacterial DNA supercoiling. This action inhibits DNA synthesis.

228 C: Higher cholesterol levels

CRP and other markers of inflammation may be elevated on presentation. They may correlate with a worse outcome. Leukocytosis may be observed within several hours after an acute myocardial infarction. It peaks in 2–4 days and returns to levels within the reference range within one week. Myoglobin is found in striated muscle. Damage to skeletal or cardiac muscle releases myoglobin into the circulation. It rises fast (within two hours) after myocardial infarction, peaks at 6–8 hours, and returns to normal in 20–36 hours. Raised d-dimer levels are also encountered early after myocardial infarction. It has no diagnostic or clear prognostic value. A lipid profile may be helpful if obtained on presentation because levels can start to drop 12–24 hours after an acute myocardial infarction. It might take several weeks before the lipid levels go back to their pre-infarction values.

229 D: Lewy body dementia

The most common cause of dementia is Alzheimer's disease, which accounts for 65% of all cases, while Lewy body dementia accounts for 7% of all cases. Dementia is a syndrome characterised by the loss of intellectual function of sufficient severity to interfere with a person's daily and occupational performance. In Lewy body dementia, in addition, two of the following three features must also be present for diagnosis: recurrent visual hallucinations (which are typically well detailed), fluctuating cognition and spontaneous motor features of parkinsonism. Supportive of the diagnosis are repeated falls, syncope, transient loss of consciousness, systematised delusions, neuroleptic sensitivity, and hallucinations in other sensory modalities. The absence of stroke, focal neurological signs and delirium makes the diagnosis of Lewy body dementia more likely.

230 B: Speech

Motor neurone disease (MND) is one of the most common neurodegenerative diseases of adult onset. Average survival from the start of symptoms is only about three years. The disease causes progressive injury and cell death of lower motor neurone groups in the spinal cord and brainstem and usually also of upper motor neurones in the motor cortex. Those affected typically develop a combination of upper and lower motor neurone signs, with progressive muscle weakness and wasting, usually accompanied by pathologically brisk reflexes and fasciculation. In patients with bulbar involvement, a mixture of spastic and flaccid components may characterise speech, resulting in a dysarthria with severe disintegration and slowness of articulation. Hypernasality occurs from palatal weakness, and patients eventually develop a strained, strangled vocal quality. With time, speech may be lost, and patients need to depend on other forms of communication, such as writing or a communication board. Most retain extra-ocular movements and bowel and bladder control. Sphincter control generally is unaffected. Because the disease primarily involves motor neurone, sensory function typically is preserved. In most patients, cognitive functioning is preserved. Remember, the three 'S's (sensation, sensorium and sphincters) are characteristically spared.

231   A: Electromyography and nerve conduction studies
The diagnosis of amyotrophic lateral sclerosis (ALS) is primarily based on the history and clinical findings. There are no specific laboratory tests to make the diagnosis. A history and physical examination, repeated at regular intervals, document progressive hyper-reflexia, fasciculation, and upper and lower motor neurone involvement. Electromyographic testing and nerve conduction studies are used for the confirmation of ALS. Diagnosis is facilitated by demonstrating diffuse denervation signs, decreased amplitude of compound muscle action potentials, and normal conduction velocities. All the other options/tests may be used to exclude alternative diagnoses.

232   D: Stop intravenous digoxin and monitor
The ventricular response rate is usually controlled with digoxin, which increases atrioventricular conduction delay and block. In paroxysmal atrial fibrillation, digoxin shortens the effective refractive period of the atrial myocardium and, if anything, would be expected to make atrial fibrillation more likely to occur and persist. The evidence available does not support a role for digoxin in suppressing recurrent AF in most patients. If he remains in sinus rhythm, no further treatment is warranted because this is the first episode of atrial fibrillation. However, if there is evidence for further recurrence a drug other than digoxin may need to be introduced.

233   A: Digoxin
Treatments for obstructive hypertrophic cardiomyopathy include medications that are negative inotropic agents, such as β-blockers and verapamil. Anti-arrhythmic drugs such as amiodarone and disopyramide are used to control arrhythmia. Positive inotropes, such as digitalis compounds, are generally avoided because of the risk of increasing the outflow obstruction in the left ventricle.

234   C: Iron and serum ferritin
Most of the other tests listed are used in ruling out reversible causes of dementia, such as depression, hypothyroidism, vitamin B_{12} and folate deficiency, neurosyphilis, subdural haematoma, brain tumour, and normal-pressure hydrocephalus. Iron deficiency or excess is not associated with dementia.

235 B: Anti-resorptive

In general, there are two classes of therapies for osteoporosis: anti-resorptive and anabolic. Anti-resorptive therapies work by reducing bone turnover, and the resulting decline results in small increases (typically 1–3%) in bone mineral density during the first year of therapy. Bisphosphonates, such as alendronate and risedronate, hormone replacement therapy, calcitonin and raloxifene (a selective oestrogen receptor modulator) are anti-resorptive while parathyroid hormone (PTH) is anabolic.

236 B: As γ-aminobutyric acid analogue

Spasticity is a central nervous system abnormality. It results from a lesion of the motor system in the brain, brainstem or spinal cord. Baclofen (Lioresa®), diazepam and dantrolene sodium (Dantrium®) are the most commonly used medications for spasticity. Baclofen, a γ-aminobutyric acid analogue, is thought to act at the spinal cord to inhibit release of excitatory neurotransmitters. Diazepam is a benzodiazepine believed to be agonistic to γ-aminobutyric acid, mostly at the spinal cord, and is primarily used in patients with spasticity of spinal cord origin. Dantrolene is a muscle relaxant and works at a different site from baclofen and diazepam, preventing calcium ion release at the sarcoplasmic reticulum and, therefore, reducing muscle contraction and spasticity. At one time it was a common choice for therapy in patients with brain injury but reports of fulminant hepatotoxicity have decreased its use.

237 A: Carcinoma of the prostate

Carcinoma of the prostate often spreads to the bones. It does not spread to the brain.

238 A: The risk of development of colon cancer is nearly 100% by the age of 40

This patient has familial polyposis coli (familial adenomatous polyposis), which involves the development of multiple adenomatous polyps, often in their hundreds. The onset of polyp formation in patients with the disease is usually after the age of 15. Colorectal carcinoma is seen, beginning 10–15 years after the onset of visible polyps The risk of development of colon cancer is nearly 100% by the age of 40. Therefore, prophylactic total colectomy is the treatment of choice.

Mucocutanous pigmentation is characteristic of Peutz–Jeghers syndrome. The polyps here are of the hamartomatous type. These usually present in early adult life and carry a low but definite risk of malignancy, probably around 5% per polyp, so they need to be excised. Peutz–Jeghers polyps can also occur in the small intestine.

239 A: Long-term proton pump inhibitor

Variceal bleeding resulting from portal hypertension is a serious complication of cirrhosis. With each incidence of bleeding, the risk of death can be as high as 50%. Patients who have had one episode of bleeding should receive secondary prophylaxis with oesophageal banding or sclerotherapy to obliterate the varices. They should also be treated with β-blockers (propranolol or nadolol) and undergo surveillance endoscopy at regular intervals. Transjugular intrahepatic portosystemic shunt (TIPS) is an effective method for reducing portal vein pressure. The indications for TIPS include uncontrollable variceal haemorrhage or recurrent variceal haemorrhage despite endoscopic therapy. Short-term proton pump inhibitors are often used with upper gastrointestinal bleeding secondary to peptic ulcer disease and upper gastrointsetinal haemorrhage induced by non-steroidal anti-inflammatory drugs. Their use in variceal bleeding is not very well supported.

240 C: Poor response to the traditional NSAIDs

Selective inhibitors of COX-2 should be used instead of standard NSAIDs only by people with rheumatoid arthritis or osteoarthritis who are at high risk of developing serious gastrointestinal adverse events. High-risk patients are defined as: those over 65 years, those already using medications known to increase the likelihood of upper gastrointestinal adverse events, those with serious co-morbidity, and those requiring prolonged use of maximum recommended doses of standard NSAIDs. If a traditional NSAID fails to produce the desired effect it can be replaced by another traditional NSAID. Selective inhibitors of COX-2 are safer but not more effective than the traditional NSAIDs.

241 A: Chest X-ray

This patient's rash in the lower limbs is typical of erythema nodosum. Sarcoidosis is only second to drug reaction as the commonest cause of erythema nodosum. A chest X-ray is therefore considered the investigation of choice. Skin biopsy will confirm the presence of vasculitic skin lesions (panniculitis) but will not help to elucidate the underlying primary cause.

242 C: Somatization disorder

This patient presents with medically unexplained symptoms (collectively known as somatoform disorders). The chronicity and large number of diverse symptoms in this case suggest somatization disorder. It is estimated that 5–10% of repeat attenders in specialist clinics have no organic pathology underlying their symptoms. The classification of medically unexplained symptoms differs between ICD-10 and DSM-IV and there is considerable overlap of syndromes. Depression is an important co-morbid (or masked presenting) disorder in this patient group. Undifferentiated somatoform disorder (single or a relatively small number of somatic complaints) appears most common, at least in primary care, with a one-year prevalence of around 14%. Conversion disorder presents with loss of function (eg paralysis) due to unconscious mechanisms. It is important to use a patient-centred, empathetic interview style with patients with somatoform disorders.

243 B: High levels are diagnostic of heart failure

Brain natriuretic peptide (BNP) is secreted in response to increased ventricular volume and pressure. Circulating BNP levels increase in proportion to the severity of the disorder, and it is detectable with minimal clinical symptoms. With a negative predictive value of greater than 95%, a normal BNP level can help exclude heart failure from other causes. Secretion of BNP from the left ventricle increases in proportion to the severity of the left ventricular dysfunction, suggesting that the secretion of BNP from the left ventricle is regulated mainly by wall tension of the left ventricle. Because conditions other than heart failure can result in an elevated BNP, the clinical context of a patient with a positive BNP must be considered. An elevated BNP level should prompt routine tests to confirm the diagnosis in addition to evaluating the cause and defining the type of heart failure (eg electrocardiography, chest X-ray and echocardiography). As for using BNP levels to monitor patients with diagnosed chronic heart failure, levels correlate well with treatment efficacy. Following an exacerbation of heart failure, a declining BNP indicates a good response to therapy and indicates a more favourable outcome. A rising BNP suggests a greater risk of adverse outcome, warranting a more aggressive treatment strategy.

244 A: Coeliac disease

Intestinal biopsies taken from individuals with coeliac disease and gluten sensitivity show a flat mucosa characterised by villus flattening and crypt elongation, with inflammatory cells in the lamina propria. The pathology is completely reversible on elimination of gluten from the diet.

245 C: Fibromyalgia

Fibromyalgia is a chronic painful disorder characterised by widespread pain in muscles and joints and excessive fatigue. Other symptoms of fibromyalgia include headache, changes in mood, difficulty in thinking and concentration, irritable bowel and urinary urgency. Physical examination often reveals multiple tender spots by applying pressure to specific locations on the neck, back, chest and limbs. The cause of fibromyalgia is not known. Laboratory markers of inflammation are characteristically normal. Fibromyalgia could either be primary where no underlying cause is identified, or secondary, when it is associated with other disorders, such as systematic lupus erythematosus and rheumatoid arthritis. Fibromyalgia is treated with non-steroidal anti-inflammatory drugs and other agents to relieve pain. Other medications can be used to help get restful sleep. A comprehensive programme of aerobic exercise, physical therapy, relaxation techniques and coping skills is beneficial for many people with this disease.

246 D: Tumour size more than 3 cm

Tumour > 3.0 cm at its greatest diameter, with no distant metastases or significant lymphadenopathy can be encountered in stage IB and IIB disease when surgery is still the treatment of choice. The A, B and C options all indicate metastatic disease. Surgery is contraindicated in patients with this level of FEV$_1$ even if the tumour is resectable.

247 D: Acute diarrhoea

Medical researchers estimate that at least half of those who seroconvert experience a 'flu-like illness at the time of initial infection. Typical symptoms include fever, headache, fatigue and enlarged lymph nodes. People may also experience aching muscles (myalgia) and a rash that occurs anywhere on the body and may change location (ie a transient generalised rash). These symptoms may last from a few days to two weeks and then subside. Oral thrush has been observed in those who have recently seroconverted. Some researchers have even reported cases of *Pneumocystis carinii* pneumonia in those newly infected. Diarrhoea is not an early feature and is usually encountered late in the disease process.

248 A: Familial periodic paralysis

Familial periodic paralysis is a condition of intermittent episodes of muscle weakness and sometimes severe paralysis. It is one of a group of genetic disorders that includes hyperkalaemic periodic paralysis, hypokalaemic periodic paralysis and thyrotoxic periodic paralysis. Thyrotoxic periodic paralysis involves attacks of muscle weakness or complete paralysis alternating with periods of normal muscle function. Attacks usually begin after symptoms of hyperthyroidism have developed. The frequency of attacks varies from daily to yearly. Episodes of muscle weakness may last for a few hours or may persist for several days. During an attack the serum potassium is low. Serum potassium levels are normal between attacks. Weakness most commonly affects the muscles of the arms and legs. It may occasionally affect the muscles of the eyes. The muscles involved in breathing and swallowing can sometimes be affected and this can be fatal. Risk factors include a family history of periodic paralysis and hyperthyroidism. Attacks may be triggered by eating high-carbohydrate or high-salt meals. Rest after vigorous exercise can also trigger an attack.

The best treatment is rapid reduction in thyroid hormone levels. Potassium should also be given during the attack. It is preferred that potassium be given by mouth, but if weakness is severe, intravenous potassium may be necessary. (NB. intravenous potassium should be given only if kidney function is adequate and if the person is monitored in a hospital.) A diet that is low in carbohydrates and salt may be recommended to prevent attacks. β-Blockers may reduce the number and severity of attacks while hyperthyroidism is brought under control. Acetazolamide is effective in attack prevention in familial periodic paralysis, but is not usually effective in thyrotoxic periodic paralysis.

249 B: Renal biopsy

Acute interstitial nephritis is an important cause of acute renal failure resulting from immune-mediated tubulo-interstitial injury, initiated by medications, infection, and other causes. Acute interstitial nephritis may be implicated in up to 15% of patients hospitalised for acute renal failure.

Renal biopsy is the gold standard for diagnosis of acute interstitial nephritis (AIN), with the typical histopathological findings of plasma cell and lymphocytic infiltrates in the peritubular areas of the interstitium, usually with interstitial oedema. Renal biopsy is not needed in all patients. In patients for whom the diagnosis seems likely, in whom a probable precipitating drug can be easily withdrawn, for example, or who improve readily after withdrawal of a potentially offending drug, supportive management can proceed safely without renal biopsy.

Renal ultrasonography may demonstrate kidneys that are normal to enlarged in size, with increased cortical echogenicity, but there are no ultrasonographic findings that will reliably confirm or differentiate AIN from other causes of acute renal failure. Gallium-67 scanning has been proposed as a useful test to diagnose AIN. The predictive value of this test is limited but it may be useful in distinguishing acute tubular necrosis from AIN. Urine eosinophils are frequently tested to provide confirmatory evidence of AIN, though the typical constellation of fever, rash, arthralgias, eosinophiluria and renal insufficiency is rarely present in its entirety. The positive predictive value of urine eosinophils is only 40%. Red cell casts are rare in AIN.

250 E: Neuroblastoma
The four most common anterior mediastinal tumours are thymomas, teratomas, lymphomas and enlarged or ectopic thyroid tissue. These are often referred to as the four 'T's (thymoma, teratoma, terrible lymphoma, and thyroid). In an adult, an upper anterior mediastinal mass (ie above the clavicles on the PA projection) which causes tracheal deviation is most likely to be of thyroid origin. Below the clavicles, thymoma is the most common. Neuroblastoma and other neurogenic tumours are often localised in the posterior mediastinum.

251 C: Ventricle (cardiac)
B-type or brain natriuretic peptide (BNP), a cardiac neurohormone, was first discovered in the brain of pigs. In humans, the main source of BNP is the ventricles of the heart.

252 C: 9-am plasma cortisol
A number of hereditary muscular dystrophies and myopathies may first show up as relatively minor symptoms, such as pain or cramping, often triggered by exercise or intercurrent illness. The major causes of an elevated creatine kinase include: metabolic disorders such as hypothyroidism, hypokalaemia, hypocalcaemia or hypomagnaesemia; inflammatory myositis (alone or as part of the spectrum of a collagen vascular disease); a paraneoplastic syndrome in malignancy; drugs (eg statins); and the hereditary myopathies/dystrophies. After a careful history, including a detailed family history, physical examination, and routine laboratory tests, the next

step should be electromyography, which will help to explain the underlying problem and to locate the optimum biopsy site. Muscle biopsy is essential in establishing the diagnosis of most inflammatory and metabolic muscle diseases. Cushing's syndrome causes myopathy and muscle weakness but the creatine kinase levels are typically normal.

253 B: Catalepsy

Catatonia is a disorder of motor activity and can occur in schizophrenia. Catalepsy, also known as waxy flexibility, is a disorder of muscle tone, which can result in patients maintaining what are often very uncomfortable postures for long periods of time without moving. Stupor, excitement and negativism are other features of catatonia. Cataplexy is the sudden loss of muscle tone. Stereotypies are repeated non-goal-directed movement (eg rocking to and fro). Mannerisms are goal-directed movements that occur out of context.

254 A: Mutation of factor V Leiden

Nephrotic syndrome is defined as proteinuria (> 3.5 g/24 h) that is sufficient to cause hypoalbuminaemia and oedema, often with hypercholesterolaemia. The cause of hypercoagulability is multifactorial in patients with nephrotic syndrome, and includes increased urinary loss of antithrombin III, altered levels and/or activity of protein C and protein S, enhanced plasma concentrations of coagulation factors, elevated von Willebrand factor, platelet hyperaggregation, depression of fibrinolysis and increased viscosity of the blood (which can be further aggravated by diuretics).

The cumulative incidence of thromboembolic complications in such patients is 50%. There are few reliable predictors of individual risk, but an albumin level lower than 25 g/l, protein excretion greater than 10 g/h, antithrombin III lower than 75% of normal, high fibrinogen levels and hypovolaemia are significantly associated with an excessive risk of thromboembolic complications. Heterozygosity for factor V Leiden is common and occurs in 5% of the general population. Patients with this disorder have a five- to ten-fold increased risk of thrombosis compared with the general population, although the risk of the first event is still low. No association between nephrotic syndrome and heterozygosity for factor V Leiden has been identified.

255 C: Benign intracranial hypertension

The normal cerebrospinal fluid (CSF) and peripheral leukocyte count make a diagnosis of chronic meningitis unlikely. Papilloedema is not associated with complicated migraine or the typical early morning headache of the sleep apnoea syndrome. Headache and blurred vision are the typical presenting symptoms of benign intracranial hypertension (pseudotumour cerebri). This condition is diagnosed by the presence of papilloedema, normal CSF (except for high pressures), normal results of diagnostic studies, and the absence of neurological defects not attributable solely to pressure. Benign intracranial hypertension was thought to be the most likely cause of this patient's symptoms. Temporal arteritis is an important consideration in patients older than 50 years who have headaches and an elevated ESR. Temporal arteritis was not considered as a cause of our patient's headaches because of her age.

256 B: Chronic alcoholism
An elevated plasma homocysteine level has been associated with upper and lower limb deep venous thrombosis, superior and inferior vena caval thrombosis, portal vein thrombosis, retinal vein and artery occlusion and coronary artery disease. Levels are higher in men and increase with age. Renal failure is also associated with elevated levels. Homocysteine rises with increasing cholesterol levels and systolic blood pressure, in smokers and in patients with vitamin B_{12} deficiency.

257 E: Renal tubular acidosis
A cerebrovascular event causing symmetrical deficits in all four limbs would be highly unlikely, and the marked electrolyte abnormalities suggest a metabolic cause for our patient's weakness. Although diuretic abuse could conceivably lead to marked hypokalaemia, a contraction alkalosis would be more likely than acidosis. Bulimia nervosa with frequent vomiting could lead to hypokalemia and poor dentition, but a metabolic alkalosis would be expected. Guillain–Barré syndrome causes symmetrical deficits in all four limbs but is not associated with hypokalaemia. Renal tubular acidosis can cause marked potassium and bicarbonate wasting in the kidneys, resulting in hypokalaemia and a high urinary pH in the setting of metabolic acidosis.

258 A: Kallmann's syndrome
Most men of reproductive age do not have a significant medical history, but some specific risk factors may be identified. For example, diabetes mellitus can cause erectile and ejaculatory dysfunction. Infertility, defined as the inability to conceive after one year of unprotected intercourse, affects 15% of couples. In the

review of systems, anosmia may suggest an underlying hypothalamic cause (such as Kallmann's syndrome) or a pituitary cause, while frequent respiratory infections are a feature of Young's syndrome (chronic sinusitis, bronchiectasis, obstructive azoospermia) and Kartagener's syndrome (primary ciliary dyskinesia/immotile cilia, chronic sinusitis, bronchiectasis, situs inversus). Headaches, visual field disturbances, or galactorrhoea should prompt an investigation for a tumour of the central nervous system.

259 D: Meningioma

Meningiomas are thought to arise from cells of the arachnoid and are usually benign, though more aggressive behaviour, characterised by repeated recurrence after surgery, is occasionally seen. Meningiomas almost always have a dural attachment. Common locations are the convexity of the cerebral hemispheres, falx cerebri, olfactory groove, sphenoid wing, cavernous sinus and tentorium cerebelli. They appear on a CT scan as a contrast-enhancing well-defined mass, often inciting a florid oedematous reaction in the brain. The overlying bone may be involved or simply thickened, producing hyperostosis.

260 E: Wernicke's encephalopathy

Wernicke's encephalopathy is caused by inadequate intake or absorption of thiamine, often in the setting of severe alcoholism. It evolves over days to weeks and has three features that may occur alone or together: abnormal eye movements, which begin with nystagmus and lateral rectus or horizontal gaze paresis and progress to complete ophthalmoplegia (the pupils are usually spared); ataxia of gait and stance, often accompanied by lower-limb intention tremor and dysmetria (the arms are usually not affected and dysarthria is usually absent); and altered mentation, the earliest signs of which are inattentiveness, mental slowing (abulia) and impaired memory. Treatment is with intravenous or intramuscular thiamine, rehydration, correction of electrolyte abnormalities, alcohol cessation and nutritional therapy. Without treatment, patients become lethargic and their condition progresses to coma and death.

Subdural haematoma is unlikely, because the patient has no history of trauma (although symptoms can occur weeks to months after an injury and in this case the patient's history may be inaccurate). Chronic subdural haematomas present weeks to months after the injury. These haematomas may become quite large without causing symptoms. The neurological findings may vary from no or minimal deficit to focal neurological symptoms that may be transient or progressive. Most patients report local back pain or radicular pain that precedes other neurological symptoms. This diagnosis is unlikely because the patient reported no pain, sensory changes, bowel incontinence, or bladder retention and he did not have a positive Babinski sign.

Central pontine myelinolysis is a demyelinating disorder that occurs most often in alcoholic or malnourished patients and is often associated with severe hyponatraemia that is iatrogenically corrected too rapidly. This diagnosis seems unlikely, because this patient's sodium derangement is minor and alcoholism has many other neurological effects that are more common. Alcohol use is known to be associated with peripheral neuropathy but this rarely affects an isolated cranial nerve. Vestibular neuronitis is often viral or idiopathic in origin.

261 B: A decrease in the proposed type II error

A is incorrect because the required sample size would decrease with an increase in the stated detectable difference.

B is correct because the power of the study is 100 (1 – type II error) %. A decrease in type II error leads to an increase in power, and an increase in power would require an increase in sample size.

C is incorrect because changes in the incidence of IBS have no effect on patients recruited to the study (who all satisfy the entry criteria of having a severe form of IBS).

D is incorrect because an increase in the significance level, say to 5%, would lead to a decrease in the required sample size.

E is incorrect because a decrease in power would lead to a decrease in the required sample size.

262 B: Hypertension

Pulse pressure is proportional to the amount of blood entering the aorta during systole and is inversely proportional to aortic compliance. Pulse pressure increases with hypertension because hypertension causes aortic compliance to decrease. Whether the hypertension is a result of an increased cardiac output or an increased peripheral resistance, the higher arterial pressure is caused by an increase in arterial blood volume. The increased blood volume stretches the arterial wall, making it stiffer and decreasing its compliance.

Stroke volume is decreased with tachycardia, haemorrhage, and heart failure, reducing pulse pressure in all three cases. In aortic stenosis the ejection of blood from the ventricle is slowed and the increase in arterial blood volume during systole is less than normal.

Causes of a widened (high) pulse pressure (> 40 mmHg), apart from isolated systolic hypertension (when it is the best blood pressure marker for cardiovascular risk), are aortic regurgitation, thyrotoxicosis, patent ductus arteriosus, arteriovenous fistula, beriberi heart, aortic coarctation and anaemia.

263 A: Chest X-ray

About 20% of patients who die of cancer have intracranial metastases. These may be solitary or multiple, and chiefly spread from primary sites in the lung (44%), breast (10%), kidney (7%), gastrointestinal tract (6%) or skin (melanoma > 3%). In 10% of cases no primary is identified. A chest X-ray therefore has the greatest chance of identifying the site of the primary cancer.

264 B: Serum albumin < 25 g/l

It is estimated that liver injury may begin to occur at a single dose of paracetamol of 15 g (30 standard tablets) or over. Indicators of severe paracetamol poisoning (ie when to contact a specialist liver centre) include: progressive coagulopathy (or INR > 2 at 24 hours, > 4 at 48 hours, > 6 at 72 hours); renal impairment (creatinine > 300 μmol/l); hypoglycaemia; metabolic acidosis (pH < 7.3, bicarbonate < 18 mmol/l) despite rehydration; hypotension despite fluid resuscitation; and encephalopathy.

265 C: Scopolamine

Various mechanisms, both peripheral and central, may play a role in the emergence of nausea and vomiting. The vomiting centre in the hypothalamus receives impulses from the chemoreceptor trigger zone (CRTZ), from cortical centres such as emotional, visual and olfactory areas, and from peripheral sources, including the inner ear and gastrointestinal tract. The CRTZ can be stimulated by chemicals, toxins, pyrogens and other endogenous substances, as well as drugs (eg digoxin, cisplatin, morphine, ipecacuanha). Dopaminergic mechanisms predominate at the CRTZ, while mainly muscarinic mechanisms operate at the vomiting centre. The choice of the most appropriate therapy for nausea and vomiting depends on the cause.

Serotonin and dopamine antagonists act centrally at the CRTZ. The best known and the prototypical serotonin ($5-HT_3$) antagonist is ondansetron. The $5-HT_3$- (5-hydroxytryptamine-3-) receptor antagonists exert their effect by blocking serotonin, both peripherally on vagal nerve terminals and centrally in the chemoreceptor trigger zone. The substituted benzamides consists of dopamine antagonists (eg metoclopramide and cisapride), which are potent anti-emetics. In addition to blocking dopamine receptors, at higher concentrations metoclopramide also blocks 5-HT$_3$ antagonists, a mechanism of action that probably contributes to its anti-emetic effects. Substituted benzamides also exert prokinetic effects on the intestine.

Cisapride is a prokinetic agent. Some phenothiazines (prochlorperazine) and butyrophenones (haloperidol) act as anti-emetics by virtue of their capacity to antagonise the action of dopamine. Atropine, scopolamine and certain anti-emetic antihistamines have prominent antimuscarinic activity and act on the vomiting centre rather than on the CRTZ.

266 B: The total daily dose of morphine should not exceed 500 mg
There is effectively no ceiling to the dose of morphine. However, if very high doses (> 1 g/day) are required, reassessment of the cause of the pain is obligatory. Anti-emetics are required in 30% of cases. A centrally acting anti-emetic (eg haloperidol or cyclizine) should be used. Opioids are seldom helpful in the management of pain resulting from muscle spasm, when diazepam and baclofen are more appropriate.

267 C: Arrange gastroscopy before starting anticoagulation
In patients taking anticoagulants, unexpected bleeding at therapeutic levels should always prompt careful assessment and investigation of the possibility of an underlying cause (eg unsuspected renal or gastrointestinal tract pathology).

268 D: Chronic myeloid leukaemia
It is becoming increasingly common for chronic myeloid leukaemia (CML) to be diagnosed by chance in patients who have no specific symptoms. Patients typically have a raised white cell count with higher than normal numbers of immature white blood cells. The count is characteristically well above normal limits and may be very high. The cells appear normal through the microscope, unlike those seen in acute leukaemia, but there are forms of blood cells that are not normally seen outside the bone marrow. The blood count and film are usually quite distinctive and the diagnosis is normally definite at this stage. A feature which tends to confirm the diagnosis is the presence of increased numbers of basophils and, to a lesser extent, eosinophils. The number of lymphocytes may be slightly elevated. In most patients there is some degree of anaemia at the time of diagnosis which is usually mild but may be severe in those patients who have been diagnosed relatively late. The platelet count is often significantly raised in chronic-phase CML and may be very high in a few patients. A bone marrow sample confirms the

diagnosis and provides important additional information. Normal bone marrow contains large numbers of fat cells with areas of blood cell production spaced between them. In CML there is very little fat present in the bone marrow, which is entirely filled with large numbers of leukaemia cells. Cytogenetic studies are of great importance, both in confirming the diagnosis of CML and in monitoring the response to treatment. The diagnosis of typical CML is confirmed in the 95% of patients who can be shown to have the *BCR-ABL* gene present (with or without the Philadelphia chromosome).

269 E: Iron is initially stored as transferrin

A well-balanced diet contains sufficient iron to meet body requirements. About 10% of the normal 10–20 mg of dietary iron is absorbed each day, and this is sufficient to balance the 1–2 mg daily losses from desquamation of epithelia. Iron is mainly absorbed in the duodenum and upper jejunum. Absorbed iron is bound in the bloodstream by the glycoprotein transferrin. Normally, about 20–45% of transferrin binding sites are filled (the percentage saturation). About 0.1% of total body iron is circulating bound to transferrin. Most absorbed iron is utilised in bone marrow for erythropoiesis. Membrane receptors on erythroid precursors in the bone marrow avidly bind transferrin. About 10–20% of absorbed iron goes into a storage pool, which is also being recycled into erythropoiesis, so there is a balance of storage and use.

The composition of the diet may also influence iron absorption. Citrate and ascorbate (in citrus fruits, for example) can form complexes with iron that increase absorption, while tannates in tea can decrease absorption. Iron homeostasis is closely regulated via intestinal absorption. Increased absorption is stimulated by decreasing iron stores, hypoxia and erythropoietic activity.

Storage iron occurs in two forms, ferritin and haemosiderin. Iron is initially stored as ferritin, but ferritin can be incorporated by phagolysosomes to haemosiderin. There are about 2 g of iron in the adult female, and up to 6 g iron in the adult male. About 1.5–2 g of this total is found in red blood cells as haem in haemoglobin, and 0.5–1 g occurs as storage iron, with the remainder in myoglobin and in enzymes that require iron.

270 A: Huntington's disease

Chorea is the most common movement disorder. In Huntington's disease (HD) chorea often appears as facial twitching or as twitching and writhing of the distal extremities. The family history is of paramount importance in making the diagnosis. If a patient with movement disorder or dementia is known to have a parent with HD, the diagnosis of HD is highly likely. Patients who develop HD by the time they are aged 35 often become bedridden within 15–20 years. Huntington's disease is an inherited disease typified by choreoathetosis, rigidity, dementia, ataxia and ophthalmoplegia. Genetically, it is an autosomal dominant disorder with complete penetrance. The mutation, CAG-trinucleotide repeats, may expand in successive generations explaining the phenomenon of anticipation. Progression is relentless, usually ending in death within 10–20 years. The CAG repeats encode glutamines in the gene for the protein 'huntingtin'. However, the role of this mutant form of huntingtin is presently unclear.

271 A: Herpes simplex encephalitis

Although the presence of fever, headache, behavioural changes, confusion, focal neurological findings and abnormal cerebrospinal fluid (CSF) findings are suggestive of herpes simplex encephalitis (HSE), no pathognomonic clinical findings reliably distinguish HSE from other neurological disorders which have similar presentations. The MRI scan shows pathological changes, which are usually bilateral, in the medial temporal and inferior frontal areas. Findings of localised temporal abnormalities are highly suggestive of HSE but confirmation of the diagnosis depends on identification of HSV within the CSF by means of polymerase chain reaction (PCR) or within brain tissue by means of brain biopsy.

272 B: Positive Babinski sign

Pain in cauda equina syndrome (CES) is often localised to the low back; local tenderness to palpation or percussion may be present, and pain in the legs (or radiating to the legs) is characteristic of CES. Reflex abnormalities may be present, typically including loss or diminution of reflexes. (Hyperactive reflexes may signal spinal cord involvement and exclude the diagnosis of CES). Sensory abnormality may be present in the perineal area or lower extremities and light touch in the perineal area should be tested. Anaesthetic areas may show skin breakdown. Muscle weakness may be present in muscles supplied by affected roots and muscle wasting may occur if CES is chronic. Poor anal sphincter tone is characteristic of CES. A positive Babinski sign or other signs of upper motor neurone involvement suggest a diagnosis other than CES, possibly a diagnosis of spinal cord compression. Alteration in bladder function may be assessed empirically by obtaining urine via catheterisation. A significant volume with little or no urge to void, or as post-void residue, may indicate bladder dysfunction.

273 C: Panic attacks
Opiate withdrawal symptoms are rarely life-threatening but can be very distressing. They can be relieved by prescribing an opiate, such as methadone, or the non-opioid lofexidine. Addiction must be confirmed prior to prescribing methadone. Features of withdrawal include rhinorrhoea and lactorrhoea, piloerection, perspiration, tachycardia, mydriasis and yawning. Although agitation occurs, panic attacks are not associated with withdrawal.

274 B: Pituitary adenoma
Cushing's syndrome is caused either by excess levels of exogenously administered glucocorticoids or by endogenous overproduction of cortisol. Endogenous glucocorticoid overproduction may be due to a primary adrenocortical abnormality (ie adenoma, carcinoma or nodular adrenal hyperplasia) or to excess adrenocorticotrophic hormone (ACTH) production. ACTH-secreting neoplasms are either an anterior pituitary tumour (Cushing's disease) or an ectopic non-pituitary tumour (eg oat cell or small cell lung carcinoma, carcinoid tumor). Ectopic corticotrophin-releasing hormone (CRH) secretion is a very rare cause of Cushing's syndrome. Of these cases, approximately 70% are caused by Cushing's disease (ie a pituitary ACTH-producing tumour), 15% to ectopic ACTH, and 15% to a primary adrenal tumor. Patients with an ACTH-producing pituitary tumour (Cushing disease) may develop headaches, visual problems, and galactorrhea. Anterior pituitary tumours may cause a rise in prolactin through compression of the pituitary stalk. Elevated prolactin levels may produce bilateral galactorrhoea that is detectable on physical examination. Other options listed are associated with cushingoid features but not with galactorrhoea.

275 C: Glucose-6-phosphate dehydrogenase (G6PD) concentration
This patient has dermatitis herpetiformis. Higher doses of dapsone are often used in this condition. Glucose-6-phosphate dehydrogenase (G6PD) deficiency is the most common human enzyme deficiency in the world, affecting an estimated 400 million people. G6PD deficiency is also known as 'favism', as G6PD-deficient people are also sometimes allergic to fava beans. G6PD deficiency is an allelic abnormality which is inherited in an X-linked recessive fashion. When someone has G6PD deficiency, complications can arise: haemolytic anaemia and prolonged

neonatal jaundice are the two major pathologies associated with G6PD deficiency. Both of these conditions are directly related to the inability of specific cell types to regenerate reduced nicotinamide adenine dinucleotide phosphate (NADPH), a reaction which is normally catalysed by the G6PD enzyme. Drugs which cause haemolysis in G6PD deficiency include dapsone and other sulphones (the higher dose used for dermatitis herpetiformis is more likely to cause problems), methylthioninium chloride (methylene blue), niridazole, nitrofurantoin, pamaquine, quinolones (including ciprofloxacin, nalidixic acid, norfloxacin, and ofloxacin), sulphonamides (including co-trimoxazole. NB. Some sulphonamides eg sulfadiazine have been tested and found not to be haemolytic in many G6PD-deficient individuals).

276 B: Causes fewer gastrointestinal side effects than the standard NSAIDs

COX-2 inhibitor drugs are as effective as traditional NSAIDs but generally cause fewer gastrointestinal effects. COX-2 inhibitors have minimal effects on platelets and can be safely given to preoperative patients and to patients with a risk of bleeding. They also can be safely given in conjunction with daily low-dose aspirin therapy. Selective COX-2 drugs offer no advantage with respect to the kidneys and should be used with care in patients with kidney dysfunction. COX-2 inhibitors, like the traditional NSAIDs, cause sodium and water retention and might necessitate an increase in antihypertensive medication in patients with hypertension.

277 E: Hyperventilation

The arterial blood gases show acute, uncompensated respiratory alkalosis. All of the options given produce this picture except acute hyperventilation. In this condition the arterial Pao_2 is increased.

278 E: Pao_2 of 8 kPa, $Paco_2$ of 8 kPa, pH 7.22

In a patient with acute hypoventilation secondary to hypnotic overdose, the pH is acidotic. Hypoxia and hypercapnia are the hallmark of type II respiratory failure encountered with hypoventilation.

279 A: Lymphoma

The presence of chyle in the pleural cavity means that there has been leakage of chyle from a damaged thoracic duct or transdiaphragmatic passage of chylous ascites. Chyle is principally derived from the lymphatic drainage of the gastrointestinal tract and contains a high concentration of triglycerides in the form of chylomicrons, which give it a milky appearance. Chylous effusions are classically painless and sterile. Neoplasms, of which most are lymphomas, account for about 50% of cases. Trauma, including cardiac surgery, accounts for about 25%. Other causes include radiotherapy, sympathectomy, birth injury, chronic pancreatitis, fibrosing mediastinitis, infections (eg lymphangioleiomyomatosis) and thoracic duct atresia. Idiopathic cases are most common in children, usually occur in boys and are right-sided. The chylous fluid is clear before the infant's first feed and cloudy thereafter.

280 C: Aortic stenosis

In a patient with heart failure the presence of atrial fibrillation, left ventricular aneurysm, left ventricular thrombus, or a history of thromboembolic disease are strong indications for anticoagulation. Aortic stenosis in the context of clinical heart failure is not in itself an indication for anticoagulation but other factors such as the degree of heart failure and mobility should be taken into consideration.

281 C: Pemphigoid

Cutaneous indications for HIV testing may be divided into strong and relative indications. Strong cutaneous indications for HIV testing include HIV exanthema, proximal subungal onychomycosis, oral hairy leukoplakia, candidiasis, molluscum on the face of an adult, Kaposi's sarcoma, bacillary angiomatosis, eosinophilic folliculitis and lipodystrophy. Relative indications for HIV testing include chronic mucocutaneous ulceration, acquired trichomegaly of the eyelashes, severe seborrhoeic dermatoses, unresponsive psoriasis and ichthyosiform dermatoses.

282 C: Decreased serum B_{12} levels

This term indicates that bone marrow erythropoiesis has a specific morphological abnormality called 'megaloblastosis'. For patients who are not on cytotoxic drugs, its presence usually indicates a deficiency of either vitamin B_{12} or folic acid. A bone marrow aspirate is not always necessary, as the presence of oval macrocytes and hypersegmented neutrophils on the blood film is strongly suggestive of its presence. A serum vitamin B_{12} and red cell folate estimation can then often make the diagnosis of folate or vitamin B_{12} deficiency. Both are needed for the normal development of haemopoietic tissue and a deficiency of either causes megaloblastic anaemia. The hypersegmentation of the nucleus is caused by defective DNA synthesis.

283 D: An increase in the central venous pressure

Veins contain the greatest percentage of blood in the body and they are very compliant. When a person stands, the combined effects of gravity and venous compliance cause blood to pool in the leg veins. Assuming a horizontal position will shift some of this blood to the vena cava because gravity no longer exerts its downward force on this volume of blood. The volume of blood that shifts into the vena cava is large enough to increase the pressure in the thoracic vena cava so that the central venous pressure will increase.

284 A: Low-dose oral steroid therapy

Primary biliary cirrhosis is a chronic liver disease that slowly destroys the bile ducts in the liver. The condition eventually leads to cirrhosis, which results in diminished liver function. The goals of treatment are to slow the progression rate of the disease and to alleviate the symptoms (eg pruritus, osteoporosis, sicca syndrome). Liver transplantation appears to be the only life-saving procedure.

Ursodeoxycholic acid is the major medication used to slow the progression of the disease. Patients with early disease show clinical, biochemical and histological improvement. Reports suggest that ursodeoxycholic acid delays the need for transplantation or delays death. The efficacy of this medication in late stages (ie cirrhosis) is questionable, however. Vitamins A, D and K are used once jaundice is present.

Pruritus is often refractory to medical therapy and has a significant impact on patients' quality of life. Antihistamines are first-line agents to relieve pruritus in the early stages and are the first line choice for patients with mild to moderate pruritus. Use caution in patients with cirrhosis and signs of encephalopathy because antihistamines can further depress brain function. Colestyramine and colestipol are effective in sequestering bile salts in the enteric lumen. A one- to four-day delay is expected before the itching remits. Corticosteroids may alleviate symptoms and improve biochemical and histological findings. However, corticosteroid-induced osteoporosis is of great concern and steroid therapy should be avoided when possible.

285 D: Behçet's disease

Scrotal ulcers, often associated with oral ulceration, venous thrombosis and inflammation of the eye is suggestive of Behçet's disease. Most of the genital ulcers in sexually transmitted disorders are painful. Genital ulcers are not a specific feature in antiphospholipid syndrome or AIDS. Primary syphilitic chancre classically presents with a single, painless indurated ulcer, which is often found on the penis.

286 B: Glomerulonephritis

This patient's skin lesion is typical of impetigo. Post-streptococcal glomerulonephritis follows group A streptococcus-induced impetigo and pharyngitis. In contrast, acute rheumatic fever follows group A streptococcus pharyngitis only. Impetigo is not one of the high-risk sources for subacute bacterial endocarditis. Furthermore, the murmur she had was not confirmed to be due to an underlying valve or other significant congenital lesion. Amoxicillin-induced rash is a well known phenomenon in patients with glandular fever. Impetigo is not associated with an increased risk of meningitis.

287 A: Serology

The diagnosis of amoebic liver abscess remains a difficult task because most of the liver function tests give non-specific results in this condition. The liver scan only showed a cold area, the cause of which cannot usually be seen. Amoebic liver abscess can be diagnosed by aspiration of the abscess, but a positive amoebic serology in a patient with a liver abscess is highly suggestive, especially if there is a history of travel, age under 50 and an acute onset. Amoebic liver abscesses often respond to medical treatment.

Routine aspiration of liver abscess is not indicated for diagnostic or therapeutic purposes. Amoebae are rarely recovered from the aspirate (15%) and often they are only present in the peripheral parts of the abscess, invading and destroying adjacent tissues. Occasionally, percutaneous diagnostic needle aspiration may be needed to differentiate between amoebic and pyogenic liver abscess. Enzyme immunoassay (EIA) has now largely replaced indirect haemagglutination (IHA) testing. The IgG EIA has a reported sensitivity of 99% and specificity greater than 90% in patients with amoebic liver abscess. Fewer than 30% of patients with amoebic liver abscess have concomitant intestinal amoebiasis so microscopic examination of stool for the identification of trophozoites or cysts is of little value. If positive, it may confirm the diagnosis. Sigmoidoscopy is rarely indicated to confirm the presence of amoebic colitis and there are no specific findings in the colon.

288 A: Carotid Doppler ultrasound

Double vision, vertigo and dysarthria are features of a brainstem lesion. This area is supplied by the vertebrobasilar vascular tree.

Imaging of the carotid arteries would have no value in assessing the posterior cerebral circulation. All of the other tests listed are appropriate and should be performed in any patient who has suffered a cerebrovascular accident, regardless of its origin.

289 E: Endocarditis

Infectious mononucleosis is characterised by the triad of fever, tonsillar pharyngitis and lymphadenopathy. A large number of other manifestations have been associated with primary Epstein–Barr virus infection, including Guillain–Barré syndrome, facial nerve palsy, meningoencephalitis, aseptic meningitis and transverse myelitis. Haematological abnormalities can include haemolytic anaemia, thrombocytopenia, aplastic anaemia and agranulocytosis. Pneumonia, myocarditis, pancreatitis and mesenteric adenitis are also reported but endocarditis is not a recognised complication.

290 A: Partial destruction of interlobular bile ducts, surrounded by mononuclear infiltrates

The histopathology of primary biliary cirrhosis (PBC) is characterised by chronic, non-suppurative, destructive cholangitis of the small interlobular bile ducts. Early lesions represent damage of the basement membrane of the bile ducts and reactive hyperplasia of the epithelial lining. Lymphocytic and plasma cell infiltration, with eosinophilic condensation in the portal tracts, is another feature. Epithelioid aggregates or granulomas may be found around the bile ducts. Fibrosis and cirrhosis develop later.

The presence of polymorphonuclear leukocytes inside the interlobular bile ducts is characteristic of acute cholangitis. Periportal plasma cell infiltration, piecemeal necrosis and bridging fibrosis are seen in patients with moderate chronic hepatitis. Epithelioid granulomas in the portal and periportal areas are often a feature of granulomatous liver diseases (eg hepatic sarcoidosis). Granuloma within the portal tract is also a feature of primary biliary cirrhosis. Liver cell necrosis, Mallory body infiltration by neutrophils and a perivenular distribution of inflammation are all typical of alcoholic liver disease.

291 A: Anti-Ro antibodies

Nearly 95% of individuals with Sjögren syndrome are ANA-positive. The principal target autoantigens are Ro (SSA) and La (SSB) antigens. The prevalence of anti-Ro antibodies varies between 40% and 95%. These are associated with the presence of extra-glandular manifestations, including vasculitis, neurological involvement,

glandular dysfunction, low haemoglobin, low total leukocyte and low platelet counts, and rheumatoid factor. Anti-La antibodies may be present in the serum of up to 87% patients with systemic sclerosis. Their presence is associated with manifestations similar to those found in anti-Ro antibodies. These two antibodies (Anti-Ro (SSA) and anti-La (SSB) antibodies) target two different ribonucleoprotein particles. They are also prevalent in patients with systemic lupus erythematosus (SLE). Anti-Ro is associated with photosensitivity, lung disease, lymphopenia and, in some cases, nephritis. Anti-La antibodies are associated with late-onset SLE, secondary systemic sclerosis, neonatal lupus erythematosus and protection from anti-Ro-associated nephritis.

292 E: Neurofibrillary tangles

The diagnosis of Alzheimer's disease is made clinically by the findings of progressive memory loss with increasing inability to participate in activities of daily living. Late in the course of the disease patients are not able to recognise family members and may not know who they are. The definitive diagnosis is made pathologically by examination of the brain at autopsy. The pathognomonic microscopic feature is an increased number of neuritic plaques in the cerebral cortex and neurofibrillary tangles (malformed nerve cells).

Axonal degeneration is one pathological form of peripheral neuropathy. It does not lead to mental changes. Loss of myelin sheaths is a feature of multiple sclerosis and other demyelinating disorders of the central nervous system and spinal cord. The clinical features of these disorders do not match this patient's presentation. A syrinx is found in the upper spinal cord and medulla oblongata in patients with syringomyelia/syringobulbia.

293 D: Oesophageal candidiasis

Candidiasis, a well-known opportunistic infection of AIDS patients, is the leading cause of infectious oesophagitis. Diagnosis of oesophageal candidiasis is usually based on the endoscopic appearance of the typical mucosal lesions and on histopathological studies. Endoscopically, patchy white plaques, confluent pseudomembrane, and friable mucosa are characteristic features of oesophageal candidiasis. Multiple raised white plaques, more than 2 mm in size, and, in the later stages, ulceration become more prominent. Nystatin or miconazole regimes can be used. Triazole drugs (eg fluconazole) should be reserved for recurrences of the disease.

Cytomegalovirus oesophagitis causes superficial erosions with serpiginous non-raised borders in the middle to distal oesophagus. With infection progression, shallow ulcerations may deepen and expand to 5–10 cm. Tissue is needed for confirmation. Similarly, herpes simplex oesophagitis begins with vesicule formation which is soon replaced by multiple small ulcers. However, an endoscopic picture of white plaque is more consistent with *Candida* infection. Histological and viral studies might prove useful in reaching the correct diagnosis in more difficult cases. Barrett's oesophagus is an erosive oesophagitis at the gastro-oesophageal junction that affects an older age group. Oesophageal webs have a different endoscopic picture.

294 D: Tick bite

Lyme disease is an illness caused by a spirochaete bacteria, *Borrelia burgdorferi*, which is transmitted to animals and man through the bite of infected ticks. *Ixodes dammini* is responsible for most of the cases of Lyme disease in the north-eastern United States. In Europe the main vector is *I. ricinus*, while *I. persulcatus* is primarily responsible for transmission in Asia. In about 50% of the cases a characteristic rash or lesion called erythema migrans is seen. It begins a few days to a few weeks after the bite of an infected tick. The rash generally looks like an expanding red ring. It is often described as looking like a bull's-eye, with alternating light and dark rings. If ignored, the early symptoms may disappear, but more serious problems can develop months to years later. The later symptoms of Lyme disease can be quite severe and chronic (arthritis, meningitis, facial palsy, heart abnormalities). These late symptoms may occur within a few weeks to months.

295 C: 45, XO

Turner's syndrome (gonadal dysgenesis) is caused by the absence of one of the sex chromosomes, monosomy of X chromosome. Cells contain only 45 chromosomes, with a single X chromosome, rather than the usual 46, XX in a female or 46, XY in a male.

XYY syndrome is a rare chromosomal disorder that affects males, caused by the presence of an extra Y chromosome. Affected individuals are usually very tall and thin. Many experience severe acne during adolescence. Other symptoms may include lower than average intelligence and antisocial or behavioural problems. Triple X syndrome is a chromosomal abnormality that affects females. No specific pattern of symptoms and malformations has been found to be associated with this abnormal chromosomal make-up.

296 E: Elevated serum urea nitrogen

There are many possible cause of pericarditis, some more common than others. In a patient with diabetes mellitus (DM) the development of kidney failure can lead to a metabolic pericarditis. DM is associated with hyperuricaemia, hypertriglyceridaemia and hypoglycaemia but these are not associated with increased incidence of pericarditis. DM is not particularly associated with hypocalcaemia.

297 C: Hepatitis C infection

Hepatocellular jaundice occurs when liver cells are damaged and unable to deal with the products of red cell breakdown. Causes of hepatocellular jaundice include the hepatitis viruses, drugs such as paracetamol (in overdose) and excessive alcohol.

In alcoholic hepatitis liver enzymes exhibit a characteristic pattern. In most patients, the AST is elevated moderately, while the ALT is normal or only mildly elevated. This is the opposite of what is observed in most other liver diseases. An AST/ALT ratio greater than 1 is almost universal in alcoholic hepatitis. Hyperbilirubinaemia in haemolysis and Gilbert's syndrome is unconjugated hyperbilirubinaemia and is usually mild. Delayed transfusion reactions are defined as haemolytic reactions occurring more than 24 hours following a transfusion of blood or blood components. In practice, most cases develop between three and thirty days after the transfusion, with an average of eight days.

298 B: Higher levels of CA 19-9 are encountered in breast cancer

CA 19-9 was initially found in colorectal cancer patients, and has also been identified in patients with pancreatic, stomach and bile duct cancer. Researchers have discovered that in those who have pancreatic cancer higher levels of CA 19-9 tend to be associated with more advanced disease. Non-cancerous conditions that may elevate CA 19-9 levels include gallstones, pancreatitis, cirrhosis of the liver and cholecystitis. CA 15-3 and CA 27-29 are elevated in breast cancer.

α-Fetoprotein (AFP) is normally produced by a developing fetus. AFP levels begin to decrease soon after birth and are usually undetectable in the blood of healthy adults (except during pregnancy). An elevated level of AFP strongly suggests the presence of either primary liver cancer or germ cell cancers of the ovary or testicle. Non-cancerous conditions that can cause elevated AFP levels include benign liver conditions, such as cirrhosis or hepatitis, ataxia telangiectasia, Wiscott–Aldrich syndrome and pregnancy.

CA 125 is produced by a variety of cells, but particularly by ovarian cancer cells. In women with ovarian cancer being treated with chemotherapy, a falling CA 125 level generally indicates that the cancer is responding to treatment. Increasing CA 125 levels during or after treatment, on the other hand, may suggest that the cancer is not responding to therapy or that some cancer cells remain in the body. Doctors may also use CA 125 levels to monitor patients for recurrence of ovarian cancer. CA 125 levels may also be elevated by cancers of the uterus, cervix, pancreas, liver, colon, breast, lung and digestive tract. Non-cancerous conditions that can cause elevated CA 125 levels include endometriosis, pelvic inflammatory disease, peritonitis, pancreatitis, liver disease and any condition that inflames the pleura. Menstruation and pregnancy can also cause an increase in CA 125.

Prostate-specific antigen (PSA) is present in low concentrations in the blood of all adult males. It is produced by both normal and abnormal prostate cells. Elevated PSA levels may be found in the blood of men with benign prostate conditions, such as prostatitis and benign prostatic hyperplasia, or with a malignant growth in the prostate. While PSA does not allow doctors to distinguish between benign prostate conditions (which are very common in older men) and cancer, an elevated PSA level may indicate that other tests are necessary to determine whether cancer is present. Improving the accuracy of PSA tests could lead to a reduction in the number of unnecessary follow-up procedures, including biopsies.

299   C: Delusions of poverty

This patient lives alone, is prescribed amitriptyline and has a previous episode of Deliberate Self Harm (DSH), suggesting she has a recent history of depression. Delusions of poverty indicate current psychotic depression (a significant risk factor for completed suicide). Approximately 10% of people with severe depression will go on to commit suicide. Previous DSH is also a significant risk factor (1% completion risk in one year), as is advancing age and poor social network. Obsessional symptoms may occur *de novo* in people with depression. Older people may have atypical presentations of depression and those presenting with attempted suicide should always have a comprehensive psychiatric assessment.

300   D: Gastric MALT lymphoma

Most cases of mucosa-associated lymphoid tissue (MALT) lymphoma affecting the stomach (approximately two-thirds) are caused by infection with *Helicobacter pylori* bacteria. Other virus/tumour associations are: human papilloma virus (HPV) with anogenital cancer/cervical cancer; Epstein–Barr virus with lymphoma; hepatitis B virus (HBV) with liver cancer; human T-cell lymphotropic virus (HTLV) with adult T-cell leukaemia; and Kaposi's sarcoma-associated herpes virus (KSHV) with Kaposi's sarcoma.

PAPER FOUR ANSWERS

301 A: Computed tomography (CT) brain scan

This patient's symptom is typical of subdural haematoma. Computed tomography is a vital tool in the assessment of patients with serious head injury and revolutionised management when it was introduced. It remains the investigation of choice even following the advent of MRI, due both to the ease of monitoring of injured patients and the better demonstration of fresh bleeding and bony injury.

The cause of a subdural haematoma is not always clear. It is probably due to trauma, often minor, in the preceding few weeks, but no such history is obtainable in 50% of cases. Symptoms are vague and often develop slowly with a gradual depression or fluctuation of consciousness. Subdural haematomas are bilateral in 10% of patients. While acute subdural haematomas show increased attenuation, this decreases with time, and they become isodense after a week or so, and hypodense thereafter. Consequently, chronic subdurals are often hypodense crescentic collections, often with mass effect. The collection may be more complex with layering of more dense material posteriorly and a gradual transition. Expansion due to osmosis may tear further veins, leading to recurrent bleeds. Hyperdense red blood cells from fresh bleeding may layer posteriorly, and complex septated collections may develop.

302 D: Exercise thallium scintigraphy

Suspected angina in a patient with left bundle branch block (LBBB) is not an infrequent scenario that we face in our clinical practice. Exercise tolerance testing will have limited value in substantiating the diagnosis or providing useful information about risk stratification and prognosis. The chronic LBBB changes will not alter during the exercise recording.

Exercise thallium-201 is injected intravenously at peak stress, and its myocardial distribution relates to coronary flow. Images are recorded with a gamma camera. This test can distinguish between reversible and irreversible ischaemia. If muscle tissue is damaged by ischaemia, it will fail to take up thallium and will be detected on the scanned image. Although it is expensive and requires specialised equipment, it is useful in patients who have left bundle branch block.

Dipyridamole-thallium scintigraphy will provide similar information to the exercise test but, whenever possible, treadmill or bicycle exercise should be used as the most appropriate form of stress because it provides the most information concerning patient symptoms, cardiovascular function and haemodynamic response during usual forms of activity. In fact, the inability to perform a bicycle or exercise treadmill test is in itself a negative prognostic factor for patients with chronic coronary artery disease.

99 mTc pyrophosphate has been used for the detection of myocardial infarction. It is used less commonly today because of the improved enzymatic detection methods for myocardial infarction. Myocardial uptake of the tracer is often seen within 10–12 hours after infarction and becomes maximal between 24 to 72 hours after infarction. The scan may remain very positive for up to six days.

A multiple gated acquisition (MUGA) scan assesses left ventricular function and can reveal salvageable myocardium in patients with chronic coronary artery disease. It can be performed with either thallium scintigraphy at rest or metabolic imaging with fluorodeoxyglucose by means of either positron emission tomography (PET) or single-photon emission computed tomography (SPECT).

303 C: Give intravenous fluids and avoid giving any antibiotics

Salmonella food poisoning is a bacterial food poisoning caused by the *Salmonella* bacterium. It results in the swelling of the lining of the stomach and intestines (gastroenteritis). While domestic and wild animals, including poultry, pigs, cattle and pets (such as turtles, iguanas, chicks, dogs and cats) can transmit this illness, most people become infected by ingesting foods contaminated with significant amounts of *Salmonella*. *Salmonella* infections usually resolve in five to seven days and often do not require treatment unless the patient becomes severely dehydrated or the infection spreads from the intestines. People with severe diarrhoea may require rehydration, often with intravenous fluids. Antibiotics are not usually necessary unless the infection spreads when it can be treated with ampicillin, gentamicin, trimethoprim/sulfamethoxazole, or ciprofloxacin. Even though *Salmonella* food poisoning is a bacterial infection, most units do not treat simple cases with antibiotics. Studies have shown that using antibiotics does not usually reduce the length of time that the patient is ill. Paradoxically, it appears that antibiotics do, however, cause the patient to shed bacteria in their faeces for a longer period of time.

304 B: Magnetic resonance imaging (MRI) of the lumbosacral region

This patient's presentation is typical of acute sciatica. It is most probably secondary to degenerative lumbar spine and intervertebral disc herniation. CT continues to be used widely in the examination of degenerative spinal disorders and excels in the evaluation of osseous features (eg osteophytes, spinal stenosis, facet hypertrophy, sclerosis) associated with degenerative disorders. MRI is the preferred procedure for evaluating intervertebral disc disease because of its superior soft tissue contrast and multiplanar capability. A focal contour abnormality of the disc margin is the hallmark of the herniated intervertebral disc. The disc fragment usually extends through a defect in the posterolateral portion of the annulus and causes compression or displacement of the ventrolateral aspect of the thecal sac, nerve roots and epidural fat. In most cases the herniated disc material is subligamentous and appears to be connected to the intervertebral portion of the disc by a narrow isthmus of tissue at the site of annular tear. This is the 'toothpaste' sign of intervertebral disc herniation.

305 C: Hepatic fibrosis

Cyclophosphamide is an alkylating cytotoxic drug. Its use is associated with nausea and vomiting. Other serious but less frequent adverse effects of this therapy include bone marrow suppression, hair loss, amenorrhoea and haemorrhagic cystitis. On rare occasions it might cause pulmonary fibrosis. Hepatic fibrosis is a recognised complication of methotrexate therapy. Treatment with cyclophosphamide is not associated with an increased risk of hepatic fibrosis.

306 C: Acute lymphoblastic leukaemia (ALL)

The presentation of significantly raised white cell count and mediastinal mass in a young adult should always raise suspicions of acute (T-cell) lymphoblastic leukaemia. T-cell ALL occurs most frequently in late childhood, adolescence and young adulthood, with a male predominance. Patients are usually males in their twenties or thirties who present with lymphadenopathy in cervical, supraclavicular and axillary regions (50%), or with a mediastinal mass (50–70%). All patients with any type of ALL will have a bone marrow sample taken to confirm the diagnosis. Sarcoidosis, Waldenström's macroglobulinaemia and lymphoma are not associated with significantly raised white cell counts. Later stages of chronic lymphatic leukaemia are associated with widespread lymphadenopathy in addition to raised white cell count. CLL is not a disease of young adults.

307 D: Carcinoma of the breast

Tobacco smoke, primarily from cigarettes, is associated with 30% of all cancer deaths in the UK. It is causally linked to cancers of the lung, upper respiratory tract, oesophagus, bladder and pancreas, and probably also a cause of cancer of the stomach, liver, kidneys, colon and rectum.

308 B: Germ cell ovarian cancer

α-Fetoprotein is a glycoprotein which is normally produced during gestation by the fetal liver and yolk sac. The serum concentration at this level is often seen in patients with hepatocellular carcinoma and tumours of gonadal origin. Elevated serum AFP occurs in pregnancy and may be seen in patients with chronic liver disease without hepatocellular carcinoma (eg in acute or chronic viral hepatitis). Adenocarcinoma of the colon and carcinoma of the head of the pancreas are associated with a rise in serum carcinoembryonic antigen and CA19 rather than AFP. Medullary carcinoma of the thyroid gland is associated with a rise in calcitonin. Serum from patients with liver cirrhosis may show increased AFP levels. The concentration of AFP is only modestly increased, however, and rarely exceeds 50 μg/l.

309 C: Coxsackie virus A

Approximately 5% of cases of possible infective endocarditis have negative blood cultures (ie culture-negative infective endocarditis). These may have non-infectious causes (eg vasculitis) or may be caused by fastidious organisms. The most common cause is the prior use of antibiotics. Fungal endocarditis always must be considered in the clinical setting of culture-negative infective endocarditis that fails to respond to appropriate antibiotic therapy. Most types of fungal infective endocarditis have a very low rate of positive blood cultures. At best, only 50% of Candida species are associated with positive blood cultures. Histoplasma and Aspergillus are almost never retrieved from the bloodstream. Serological tests are helpful for diagnosing valvular infection with fastidious organisms (eg, Coxiella burnetii and Chlamydia, Brucella and Legionella species). Coxsackie virus A is rarely associated with infective endocarditis or vegetations.

310 D: Bone marrow biopsy

This patient's clinical presentation suggests a diagnosis of pancytopenia, which could either be due to aplastic anaemia or to another bone marrow disorder, such as infiltration, drugs or an autoimmune disorder. To diagnose aplastic anaemia there must be at least two of the following: haemoglobin < 10g/dl, platelet count < 50 x 10⁹/l, neutrophil count < 1.5 x 10⁹/l. Patients with aplastic anaemia most commonly present with symptoms of anaemia and skin or mucosal haemorrhage or visual disturbance due to retinal haemorrhage. Infection is a less common presentation. The absent lymphadenopathy and hepatosplenomegaly strongly suggest the diagnosis of aplastic anaemia. Their presence would suggest another diagnosis.

Both a bone marrow aspirate and trephine biopsy are required to establish the diagnosis and exclude other alternative possibilities. Aplastic anaemia is defined as pancytopenia with a hypocellular bone marrow in the absence of an abnormal infiltrate and with no increase in reticulin. Erythropoiesis is reduced or absent. Megakaryocytes and granulocytic cells are reduced or absent. Lymphocytes, macrophages, plasma cells and mast cells appear prominent. A trephine is crucial to assess overall cellularity, to assess the morphology of residual haemopoietic cells and to exclude an abnormal infiltrate. In most cases the trephine is hypocellular throughout.

311   B: Down's syndrome
This karyotype corresponds to a female with an extra chromosome 21, typical of Down's syndrome.

312   E: Heterozygotes are rarely clinically affected
Heterozygotes for familial hypercholesterolaemia have elevated levels of LDL cholestrol from birth and are at an increased risk of atherosclerotic coronary heart disease at a younger age than normal.

313   C: Suppression of δ-aminolaevulinic acid (ALA) synthetase activity
In acute intermittent porphyria the increased activities of ALA synthetase is thought to be due to decreased feedback inhibition due to the primary block in haem synthesis, ie uroporphinogen synthetase. Following the adminstration of haematin, there is immediate feedback inhibition of ALA synthetase with a subsequent decrease in ALA and porphobilinogen synthesis.

314   A: Flecainide
Flecainide is a class IC anti-arrhythmic drug that blocks sodium channels and slows cardiac conduction. Flecainide is used to treat a variety of arrhythmias, including atrial fibrillation, supraventricular tachycardia and ventricular premature beats. Flecainide has a negative inotropic effect and is better avoided in congestive heart failure. The Cardiac Arrhythmia Suppression Trial (CAST) is a long-

term multicentre randomised study of patients with ventricular arrhythmia and acute myocardial infarction. It was found that flecainide increased the mortality of patients in this trial compared to placebo. Because of the findings of the CAST trial, flecainide's use has been restricted primarily to treating atrial fibrillation and other supraventricular arrhythmias in patients without evidence of prior heart attack and in whom the risk of heart attack is thought to be low.

315 B: Selective IgA deficiency

Selective IgA deficiency is the most common primary immune deficiency syndrome. It is associated with increased infections of the respiratory and gastrointestinal tracts and an increased incidence of atopy. Severe reactions to infusion of blood products have been reported. C1 esterase inhibitor deficiency is associated with angioneurotic oedema which not related to blood infusion. Hyperimmunoglobulinaemia IgE syndrome is associated with increased incidence of staphylococcal abscess formation. It is not particularly caused by or associated with an allergic reaction. Adenosine deaminase deficiency is associated with combined cellular and humoral immunodeficiency. Patients with DiGeorge's syndrome have cellular immunodeficiency.

316 B: Peripheral vascular resistance

Although an increase in cardiac output can contribute to an increase of blood pressure, the arteriolar vascular resistance is by far the most important determinant of blood pressure. The other three factors mentioned are determinants of cardiac output and are therefore not primary factors in modulating blood pressure.

317 C: Bilateral sacroiliitis

Pain and prolonged stiffness in the low back in a young adult is highly suggestive of ankylosing spondylitis. The onset is usually gradual and progressively worsens over several months. The symptoms of pain and stiffness are often worse in the morning, or after prolonged periods of inactivity, and are often eased by movement, heat and a warm shower in the morning. The disease typically starts at the sacroiliac joint and spreads upwards. Bilateral sacroiliitis can be identified in more than 50% of established cases. Ossification spreads upwards within the longitudinal ligaments and the fibrocartilaginous ring of the intervertebral disc forms syndesmophytes (radiodense lines that connect vertebrae). With enough syndesmophyte formation, the whole spine develops an undulating contour called 'Bamboo Spine'.

Disc space narrowing and osteophyte formation are features of degenerative spine disorders (lumbar spondylosis). Normal radiographic findings can be obtained very early in the disease. However, early symptoms in a young fit male are often attributed to mechanical or sports injury and therefore most patients' presentation is delayed and they are often seen with established disease and a greater chance of positive spine X-rays.

318　D: Knee reflex

Clinical tests for absent brainstem reflexes show:

- No pupillary response to light
- Absent corneal reflex
- No motor response within cranial nerve distribution
- Absent gag reflex
- Absent cough reflex
- Absent vestibulo-ocular reflexes.

319　E: Lymphadenopathy is the most common abnormal finding on chest X-rays

More than 90% of patients have characteristic but non-specific thoracic lymphadenopathy which is visible on chest X-rays. Bilateral symmetrical hilar adenopathy presents in the majority of cases. Serum angiotensin-converting enzyme (ACE) is thought to arise in vascular endothelial cells. Serum ACE is commonly elevated in sarcoidosis, but this elevation is both non-specific and insensitive. A definitive diagnosis requires the histological identification of non-caseating granulomas. Histology by itself, however, is not sufficient to make the diagnosis of sarcoidosis because a variety of infections and other diseases, including malignancies, are also associated with non-caseating granulomas. Pulmonary function studies can be normal initially. If the disease is more advanced, abnormalities associated with interstitial lung disease are found. Most patients have restrictive lung disease but endobronchial granulomas can also result in an element of airway obstruction.

320　A: Pseudogout

Pseudogout often occurs suddenly and tends to strike the knees or wrists. Episodes frequently occur following surgery, trauma or major medical illness. Attacks of pseudogout are usually monoarticular, but two or more joints may be involved simultaneously. Joint aspiration would establish the diagnosis. A rod or rhomboid crystal with weakly positive birefringence in the synovial fluid is the hallmark of pseudogout. Gout is more likely to strike the big toe or the foot. Septic arthritis is very unlikely to present in more than one joint. Abrupt knee swelling would be an unusual presentation for rheumatoid arthritis or osteoarthritis.

321 D: Receptive dysphasia

Haemorrhage into the pons (usually the result of hypertensive vascular disease) results in coma (from involvement of the reticular formation), decerebrate posturing (lesions between the red nucleus and the vestibular nucleus), small pupils (involvement of descending sympathetic fibres) and quadraplegia. It is sometimes associated with a high temperature. Dysphasia is not a feature of pontine haemorrhage because the bleeding originates from the posterior cerebral circulation and not from the carotid circulation.

322 C: Superior mesenteric angiography

The clinical and laboratory findings are highly suggestive of insulinoma. The diagnostic efforts should be directed towards localising the tumour using such techniques as ultrasound, computed tomography, arteriography and selective pancreatic venous catheterisation.

323 B: Osteopenia

Hypogonadism frequently accompanies hyperprolactinaemia and is often manifested clinically by amenorrhoea and/or other ovulatory disorders. Because mean serum oestradiol levels in amenorrhoeic hyperprolactinaemic women are typically comparable to the early follicular phase oestradiol levels seen in normal women, hyperprolactinaemic amenorrhoeic women have an absolute or relative oestrogen deficiency state. Such women lack the rise in serum oestradiol levels typically seen in the mid-follicular, ovulatory and luteal phase of the cycle. The long-term metabolic consequences of amenorrhoea and its associated oestrogen deficiency in young women have been the subject a number of studies. Osteopenia has been found to affect both cortical and trabecular bone compartments and progressive cortical and trabecular bone loss has been demonstrated in untreated patients. Acanthosis nigricans and excessive perspiration are features often seen in acromegaly. Hyperprolactinaemia is not associated with arthritis and hyperpigmentation.

324 D: Oral contraceptive pills

Elevated serum prolactin levels can occur secondary to a wide variety of factors. In addition to prolactin-secreting adenoma, numerous drugs, such as oral contraceptive pills, phenothiazines and opiates, can induce hyperprolactinaemia. Hypothyroidism, cirrhosis and renal failure are also known to be associated with high levels of prolactin. Central nervous system disorders such as sarcoidosis, epileptic fits or trauma that results in stalk section that interferes with the portal blood flow can lead to hyperprolactinaemia. Therefore it is important not to assume that an elevated prolactin level necessarily indicates the presence of a prolactin-secreting pituitary tumour.

325 E: pH 7.30, Paco$_2$ 8.0 kPa, bicarbonate 26 mmol/l

This patient has compensated chronic respiratory acidosis due chronic obstructive pulmonary disease.

Interpretation of acid–base disorders:

- Acidosis (pH < 7.4)
  with a low bicarbonate (< 24 mmol/l) = metabolic
  with a high Paco$_2$ (> 6 kPa) = respiratory
- Alkalosis (pH > 7.4)
  with a high bicarbonate (> 24 mmol/l) = metabolic
  with a low Paco$_2$ (< 6 kPa) = respiratory

Compensation (a chronic response) has occurred in:

- Metabolic acidosis if the Pco$_2$ is low (< 6 kPa)
- Respiratory acidosis if the bicarbonate is high (> 24 mmol/l)
- Metabolic alkalosis if the Pco$_2$ is high (> 6 kPa)
- Respiratory alkalosis if the bicarbonate is low (< 24 mmol/l).

326 E: The plasma volume is 3 litres

Water distribution in a 60 kg individual:

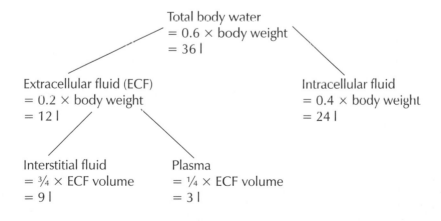

Total body water
= 0.6 × body weight
= 36 l

Extracellular fluid (ECF)
= 0.2 × body weight
= 12 l

Intracellular fluid
= 0.4 × body weight
= 24 l

Interstitial fluid
= ¾ × ECF volume
= 9 l

Plasma
= ¼ × ECF volume
= 3 l

327 A: Atrial septal defect

In non-prosthetic valve endocarditis, the proportion of males is higher than females, and most patients are over the age of 50. Endocarditis is uncommon in children. Between 60% and 80% of patients have an identifiable predisposing cardiac lesion. Rheumatic valvular disease accounts for about 30% of cases. The mitral valve is most commonly involved, followed by the aortic. Right-sided endocarditis usually affects the tricuspid valve but is rare on rheumatic valves. Congenital heart disease other than mitral valve prolapse is the underlying lesion in around 10–20% of patients with endocarditis. Predisposing lesions include patent ductus arteriosus, ventricular septal defect, tetralogy of Fallot, coarctation of the aorta, pulmonary stenosis and bicuspid aortic valve but not uncomplicated atrial septal defect. Mitral valve prolapse is the underlying lesion in around 10–33% of cases.

328 A: Growth hormone

Growth hormone-secreting cells are acidophilic in nature. The association of acidophilic tumours with acromegaly has linked these cells to the production of growth hormone. TRH is released by the hypothalamus; the anterior pituitary secretes thyroid-stimulating hormone (TSH). TSH-secreting cells produce a glycoprotein hormone and consequently are basophilic, showing positive PAS staining. Gonadotrphic hormones (FSH and LH) are secreted by basophilic cells. ACTH-secreting cells are basophilic cells which are derived embryologically from the intermediate lobe.

329 E: Increased contractility of the heart

Inotropic effects are ones that change the strength of contraction of the heart muscle. A positive inotropic drug will increase cardiac muscle contractility and a negative inotropic drug will decrease it.

330 A: Increase in the number of mitochondria per muscle fibre

The mitochondria are the aerobic energy factories of cells. Long runs increase the number and size of the mitochondria in muscle fibres. With more mitochondria, more energy can be produced aerobically and a faster pace can be maintained. Enzymes in the mitochondria speed up aerobic energy production. Long runs increase the activity of these enzymes and therefore also improve the efficiency of the mitochondria.

331 E: Interleukin-4
Th1 cells produce the inflammatory cytokine interferon-γ (IFN-γ), which activates intracellular killing mechanisms in macrophages, promotes cellular immunity, and is the appropriate response to intracellular pathogens such as *Listeria monocytogenes*. In contrast, Th2 cells produce the cytokine interleukin-4 (IL-4), which enhances B cell development and promotes humoral immunity.

332 C: Paternal age
The frequency of this mutation increases two- to three-fold after paternal age > 40. There is a strong paternal age effect for many but not all dominant mutations. Fortunately, most of these are rare.

333 A: Chelate calcium
The citrate ion has three anionic carboxylate groups that avidly chelate calcium and reduce the concentration of free calcium in blood. Because free calcium is required for multiple steps in both coagulation pathways, citrate is a useful in-vitro anticoagulant.

334 B: Cause a decrease in the ozone layer
CFCs are a family of chemicals containing chlorines and fluorines used as refrigerants and in the manufacture of many products from foam insulation to computer chips. Of the CFCs in the atmosphere 3.1% come from aerosol sprays, 27.5% from foams, 16.2% from automotive air conditioning, 15.6% from refrigeration and air conditioning and 12% from halon fire extinguishers. Industries are now beginning to successfully find alternatives to CFCs. CFCs have been banned for many uses in the US, but are still being used internationally. They are released to the atmosphere, where they drift around and eventually make it up to the stratosphere. In the atmosphere, sunlight causes them to break down, releasing chlorine. The chlorine ions combine with ozone, forming a compound called chlorine dioxide and freeing one of ozone's oxygen atoms. The chlorine dioxide then breaks up, and the chlorine ion continues to knock out one oxygen atom after another from a whole series of ozone molecules. Partially because of the CFCs in the atmosphere, the ozone layer has been depleted at the rate of about 4–5% over the last decade. This is already making its mark – it has been estimated, for example, that two out of three Australians will have skin cancer by the age of 70. This would be due to the decrease in the ozone layer and the resulting lack of absorption of ultraviolet rays.

335 D: Sampling from the 'drip' arm

This is the typical result of sampling from the 'drip' arm in a patient receiving 5% dextrose. Note that the blood is still iso-osmolar – in contrast to most of the 'real' causes of extreme hyponatraemia (eg SIADH, adrenal insufficiency and hypothyroidism). All of such cases of hyponatraemia are associated with a low plasma osmolality. The normal ECG and normal cardiac enzymes are against the diagnosis of acute myocardial infarction.

336 C: Mobitz type II second-degree AV block

The recommendations for the institution of temporary transvenous pacing, from class 1 (most pursuasive) to class 3 (least pursuasive) are:

Class 1

- Asystole
- Symptomatic bradycardia (includes sinus bradycardia with hypotension and type I second-degree AV block with hypotension not responsive to atropine)
- Bilateral BBB (alternating BBB or RBBB with alternating LAFB/LPFB) (any age)
- New or indeterminate age bifascicular block (RBBB with LAFB or LPFB, or LBBB) with first-degree AV block
- Mobitz type II second-degree AV block.

Class 2a

- RBBB and LAFB or LPFB (new or indeterminate-age)
- RBBB with first-degree AV block
- LBBB, new or indeterminate
- Incessant VT, for atrial or ventricular overdrive pacing
- Recurrent sinus pauses (greater than three seconds) not responsive to atropine.

Class 2b

- Bifascicular block of indeterminate age
- New or age-indeterminate isolated RBBB.

Class 3

- First-degree heart block
- Type I second-degree AV block with normal haemodynamics
- Accelerated idioventricular rhythm
- Bundle branch block or fascicular block known to exist before acute MI.

(Where BBB = bundle branch block; RBBB = right bundle branch block; LBBB = left bundle branch block; LAFB = left-anterior fasicular block; LPFB = left-posterior fasicular block; AV = atrioventricular; VT = ventricular tachycardia.)

337 C: Rheumathoid arthritis

HLAs (human leukocyte antigens) are proteins present in the cell membranes of nearly every cell in the body (all nucleated cells). These antigens are in especially high concentrations on the surface of white blood cells (leukocytes). HLAs are the major determinants used by the body's immune system for recognition and differentiation of self from non-self. Many HLA molecules exist but some are of special interest because they are more common in certain autoimmune diseases. For example, HLA-B27 is found in 80–90% of people with ankylosing spondylitis and can aid in the diagnosis of this disease. However, HLA-B27 is also present in 5–7% of people without autoimmune disease. Thus, the mere presence of this HLA molecule is not indicative of disease by itself. However, lack of HLA-B27 virtually excludes ankylosing spondylitis. Similarly the lack of HLA-DR2 (HLA-DQB1*0602) excludes narcolepsy. The presence of HLA-DR4 serves to delineate a subgroup of patients with rheumatoid arthritis with a poorer prognosis. Haemochromatosis is strongly associated with HLA-A3 but recent data has confirmed that another gene is involved in this disease, namely *HFE*, which is closely linked to the gene for HLA-A3 but is in fact a different gene. Beçhet's disease is associated with HLA-B51.

330 D: K^+

	Concentration in extracellular fluid (mmol/l)	Concentration in intracellular fluid (mmol/l)
Na^+	145	12
K^+	4	150
Ca^{2+}	5	0.001
Chloride	105	5
Bicarbonate	24	12
Phosphate	2	100

There is unequal distribution of Na^+ and K^+ in extracellular and intracellular fluids as a result of membrane-bound Na^+K^+-ATPase.

339 B: Typical claw-hand deformity

Complete ulnar paralysis results in a characteristic claw-hand deformity owing to wasting and weakness of many of the small hand muscles and hyperextension of the fingers at the metacarpophalangeal joints and flexion at the interphalangeal joints. The flexion deformity is most pronounced in the fourth and fifth fingers. Sensory loss occurs over the fifth finger, the ulnar aspect of the fourth finger, and the ulnar border of the palm. The superficial location of the nerve at the elbow makes it a common site for pressure palsy. The ulnar nerve may also become entrapped just distal to the elbow in the cubital tunnel formed by the aponeurotic arch linking the two heads of the flexor carpi ulnaris. Also, prolonged pressure on the base of the palm, as occurs with the use of hand tools or bicycle riding, may result in damage to the deep palmar branch of the ulnar nerve, causing weakness of the small hand muscles but no sensory loss. Valgus deformity at the elbow is often associated with ulnar nerve injury.

340 E: Recommending no further follow-up

A cervical bruit is not necessarily indicative of carotid stenosis. Neck bruits do not reliably predict the presence or absence of underlying occlusive carotid disease. Cervical bruits may be due to other causes, such as transmitted cardiac murmurs, anatomical variations, tortuosity, and hyperdynamic states. Patients with asymptomatic bruits are less likely to have an underlying stenosis than patients with symptomatic bruits (ie associated with cerebrovascular accident or transient ischaemic attack). Furthermore, the treatment of asymptomatic carotid stenosis is not well established and is still controversial. The lack of symptoms, the patient's relatively young age and the absence of any risk factor renders the likelihood of critical carotid stenosis very remote. The best option at this stage is probably to reassure and recommend no further follow-up in the near future.

341 D: It is more common in women than in men

A dry, tickly and often bothersome cough is the most common adverse effect of ACE inhibitors. Recent studies indicate that cough may develop in around 10% of the patients treated with ACE inhibitors. In half of these patients, the ACE inhibitor has to be discontinued. Cough has emerged as a class effect, occurring with all ACE inhibitors with no clear difference between the single substances. While ACE inhibition is safe in the vast majority of patients with obstructive airways disease, asthmatic symptoms or exacerbation of asthma, as well as a rise in bronchial reactivity, have occasionally been reported. ACE inhibition increases the cough reflex.

The mechanisms underlying ACE inhibitor-induced cough are probably linked to suppression of kininase II activity, which may be followed by an accumulation of kinins, substance P and prostaglandins. Physicians should be aware that a dry cough is the most common adverse effect of ACE inhibitors and that this symptom may not necessarily occur shortly after institution of therapy but months or even a year later. Replacement by another ACE inhibitor should not be tried as the cough will almost always recur on re-challenge with the same or another ACE inhibitor. After withdrawal of the ACE inhibitor, which is the treatment of choice, cough will usually resolve within a few days. This cough occurs more commonly in women than in men.

342   D: The serum erythropoietin is low

Typically, patients present with an elevated haemoglobin concentration and haematocrit, associated with thrombocytosis, leukocytosis and splenomegaly. Determination of the serum erythropoietin concentration is important in distinguishing primary from secondary causes of polycythaemia. An elevated erythropoietin concentration suggests secondary erythrocytosis, while a low level is compatible with PRV. In PRV, the neutrophil alkaline phosphatase score is frequently increased, as is the serum vitamin B_{12} level and serum vitamin B_{12}-binding capacity. Splenomegaly is often identified on physical examination but lymphadenopathy is not a recognised feature of PRV.

343   C: It acts in the terminal ileum

Intrinsic factor is a glycoprotein secreted by parietal cells of the gastric mucosa. It has an important role in the absorption of vitamin B_{12} (cobalamin) in the intestine, and failure to produce or utilise intrinsic factor results in pernicious anaemia. Dietary vitamin B_{12} is released from ingested proteins in the stomach through the action of pepsin and acid. It is rapidly bound by one of two vitamin B_{12}-binding proteins that are present in gastric juice. At acid pH these binding proteins have a greater affinity for the vitamin than does intrinsic factor. In the small intestine, pancreatic proteases digest the binding proteins, releasing vitamin B_{12} which then becomes bound to intrinsic factor. Finally, there are receptors for intrinsic factor on the ileal mucosa which bind the complex, allowing vitamin B_{12} to be absorbed into the portal blood.

Since efficient absorption of vitamin B_{12} in humans depends on intrinsic factor, diseases which decrease the secretion of intrinsic factor (eg atrophic gastritis) interfere with cleavage of the binding proteins (eg pancreatic exocrine insufficiency) or decrease binding and absorption of the intrinsic factor–vitamin B_{12} complex (eg ileal disease or resection) can result in this type of anaemia.

344 A: It appears as extracellular basophilic hyaline material

Amyloidosis is the deposition of an extracellular basophilic hyaline material in the body. Methotrexate does not cause amyloidosis or nephrotic syndrome. Congo red staining shows green birefringence by polarising microscopy, specific and unique properties shared by all amyloids due to their β-pleated fibrillar structure. Systemic amyloidosis (AA amyloid) related to chronic inflammation (eg rheumatoid arthritis) tends to involve parenchymatous organs, such as the kidneys, spleen, liver and adrenals, while amyloidosis related to myeloma (AL amyloid) tends to affect mesodermal or other tissues, such as the heart, gastrointestinal tract, peripheral nerves, skin and tongue.

345 A: Reduces body fat

Leptin (from the Greek *leptos*, meaning thin) is a protein hormone with important effects in regulating body weight, metabolism and reproductive function. Leptin is expressed predominantly by adipocytes, which fits with the idea that body weight is sensed as the total mass of fat in the body. Leptin's effects on body weight are mediated through effects on hypothalamic centres that control feeding behaviour and hunger, body temperature and energy expenditure. Decreased hunger and food consumption is mediated at least in part by inhibition of neuropeptide Y synthesis. Neuropeptide Y is a very potent stimulator of feeding behaviour. The second main effect of leptin is increased energy expenditure, measured as increased oxygen consumption, higher body temperature and loss of adipose tissue mass. Daily injections of recombinant mouse or human leptin into ob/ob mice (ie obese mutants unable to synthesise leptin) led to a dramatic reduction in food intake within a few days, and to roughly a 50% reduction in body weight within a month.

346 E: Hypothermia

Pulse oximetry is a simple non-invasive method of monitoring the percentage of haemoglobin which is saturated with oxygen. The pulse oximeter consists of a probe attached to the patient's finger or ear lobe which is linked to a computerised unit. The oxygen saturation should always be above 95%. An oximeter detects hypoxia before the patient becomes clinically cyanosed. A source of light originates from the probe at two wavelengths (660 nm and 940 nm). The light is partly absorbed by haemoglobin, by amounts which differ depending on whether it is saturated or desaturated with oxygen. By calculating the absorption at the two wavelengths the processor can compute the proportion of haemoglobin which is oxygenated. The oximeter depends on a pulsatile flow and produces a graph of the quality of flow. Where flow is sluggish (eg in hypovolaemia or vasoconstriction) the pulse oximeter may be unable to function.

In a number of situations the pulse oximeter readings may not be accurate. The presence of abnormal haemoglobins, as in methaemoglobinaemia (eg following an overdose of prilocaine), causes readings to tend towards 85%. Carboxyhaemoglobin (carbon monoxide poisoning) causes saturation values to tend towards 100%. A pulse oximeter is extremely misleading in cases of carbon monoxide poisoning for this reason and should not be used. CO-oximetry is the only available method of estimating the severity of carbon monoxide poisoning. Dyes and pigments, including nail varnish, may give artificially low values. Vasoconstriction and hypothermia cause reduced tissue perfusion and failure to register a signal.

Rare cardiac valvular defects (eg tricuspid regurgitation) cause venous pulsation and therefore venous oxygen saturation is recorded by the oximeter. Oxygen saturation values less than 70% are inaccurate as there are no control values to compare them with. Cardiac arrhythmias may interfere with the oximeter picking up the pulsatile signal properly and with calculation of the pulse rate.

Age, sex, anaemia, jaundice and skin colour have little or no effect on oximeter function.

347 E: Haemorrhage
This clinical picture is consistent with pump failure or right ventricular outflow obstruction. In haemorrhage the central venous pressure (CVP) is low.

348 A: Intubation and positive-pressure ventilation
The diagnosis is a pneumothorax. If he is in extremis time should not be wasted on performing a chest X-ray and immediate decompression with a needle should be performed. Intermittent positive-pressure ventilation (IPPV) may worsen the pneumothorax if it is not decompressed first.

349 E: Increased muscular efficiency at high blood lactate levels
Cardiorespiratory adaptions in athletes at rest are:

- Increased heart size
- Increased stroke volume
- Lower resting heart rate
- Stable cardiac output
- An increased total blood volume
- Increased parasympathetic activity
- Decreased blood pressure
- Increased muscular efficiency at high blood lactate levels.

350 A: Absent knee tendon jerk
This patient has backache with radiation to the anterior thigh. He also has weakness in the hip flexors and probably the quadriceps as well. High lumbar disc herniation (L2, L3, or L4) root or femoral nerve lesion is the most likely cause behind this patient's complaint. The knee jerk may be diminished or absent. Quadriceps atrophy and weakness may be found. The reverse straight leg raising test often reproduces the back and anterior thigh pain. It can be tested by flexing the knee with the patient prone, which may reproduce the back and anterior thigh pain. The sciatic nerve originates in the sacral plexus, mainly from the L5–S2 spinal segment. It supplies muscles that cause extension of the thigh and flexion of the leg. It is responsible for all foot movements. Therefore, pain usually radiates down the posterior and lateral leg, to below the knee. Foot-drop and positive straight leg raising are features suggestive of L5/S1 root lesion.

351 E: The difference is statistically significant at the 5% level
A is inappropriate because it is not possible to say anything about the actual difference from the information given in the question
B is inappropriate because no information on the actual survival proportions is given
C is inappropriate because a statistically significant difference between the survival proportions was found and no information on the actual survival proportions is given
D is incorrect because a statistically significant difference between the survival proportions was found, hence it is unlikely to have arisen by chance
E is correct because if $p < 0.01$ then it follows that $p < 0.05$

352 C: Ulcerative colitis

Hypertrophic osteoarthropathy (HOA) is a syndrome characterised by proliferative changes in the skin and skeleton. Proliferative periostitis of the radius and fibula and digital clubbing are commonly seen. Two forms of the syndrome are seen, a rare idiopathic from called 'pachydermoperiostitis' (3–5%), a familial autosomal dominant condition, and a more common secondary form (95–97%). Secondary HOA was initially described in association with chronic suppurative infection and malignancy of the lung and pleura. It therefore used to be called 'hypertrophic pulmonary osteoarthropathy' (HPOA). Pleural causes include pleural fibroma and mesothelioma. Pulmonary causes include bronchogenic carcinoma; pulmonary tuberculosis; pulmonary abscesses; bronchiectasis; emphysema; and *Pneumocystis carinii* infection in patients with AIDS, Hodgkin's disease, metastases, or cystic fibrosis. Cyanotic heart disease with a right-to-left shunt is the only cardiac cause described. Abdominal causes include liver cirrhosis, ulcerative colitis, Crohn's disease, Whipple's disease and biliary atresia. In long-standing insulin-dependent diabetes mellitus, contracture of the flexor tendons of the fingers with a tight, waxy skin appearance leads to diabetic cheirarthropathy. There is no pain and minor functional impairment. Neither diabetes mellitus nor any inflammatory arthritis is associated with HOA.

353 C: Thyroid function tests

Pseudogout accurately describes acute attacks of CPPD crystal-induced synovitis which clinically resemble urate gout. However, the majority of individuals with CPPD crystal deposition never experience such episodes. 'Chondrocalcinosis' is the term used to describe the calcium-containing deposits that are found in cartilage and which are usually visible on joint X-rays. A variety of metabolic and endocrine disorders are associated with CPPD crystal deposition, including haemochromatosis, Wilson's disease, hypothyroidism, hyperparathyroidism, hypomagnesaemia and hypophosphatasia.

354 C: Reflex sympathetic dystrophy

Reflex sympathetic dystrophy is a pain syndrome caused by a dysfunction of the autonomic nervous system. It is generally caused by some trauma such as an accident or surgery. However, it may occur without apparent injury. This disease normally begins in one hand or foot. Sadly, it tends to progress with time to other parts of the body. Furthermore, rather than getting less painful, as the disease progresses it can become more painful. Patients have described it as walking around with a nail stuck in your foot, or with your hand inside a glove filled with caustic acid. The pain is intense and burning, and is not significantly reduced by normal pain medication. One visible sign of reflex sympathetic dystrophy near the site of injury is warm, shiny red skin that later becomes cool and bluish. The pain that patients report is out of proportion to the severity of the injury and gets worse, rather than better, over time. Eventually the joints become stiff from disuse, and the skin, muscles and bone atrophy.

355   B: Intravenous lorazepam

Continuous seizures, or two or more seizures occurring in sequence without recovery of consciousness between them is, by definition, status epilepticus. Convulsive status epilepticus is an emergency that is associated with high morbidity and mortality. The outcome largely depends on the cause, but prompt and appropriate pharmacological therapy can reduce morbidity and mortality. Immediate concerns include supporting respiration, maintaining blood pressure, gaining intravenous access and identifying and treating the underlying cause. Initial therapeutic and diagnostic measures are conducted simultaneously. The goal of therapy is rapid termination of clinical and electrical seizure activity; the longer a seizure continues, the greater the likelihood of an adverse outcome. Several drug protocols now in use will terminate status epilepticus. Lorazepam (0.1 mg/kg) by slow intravenous push as initial therapy in patients with status epilepticus is the drug of choice. If clinical or electrical evidence of seizure activity persists, switch to phenytoin 20 mg/kg or the equivalent of phosphenytoin. The dose should be increased by increments of 5 mg/kg up to a total of 30 mg/kg if necessary. An alternative approach, when the initial lorazepam infusion fails, is to go directly to intubation and general anaesthesia.

356   E: Supraspinatus tendonitis

The information given indicates that the supraspinatus tendon is inflamed. The results of the motion tests, and especially the location of pain on palpation, are the key indicators suggesting supraspinatus tendonitis. The pain from abduction against resistance results directly from the action of the supraspinatus muscle, which initiates abduction. The pain felt between 70° and 120° with no resistance is probably due to compression of the supraspinatus tendon between the greater tubercle of the humerus and the acromion process. Abduction of the arm is actually a fairly complex process. During the first 30° of abduction, only the glenohumeral joint is in motion, caused first by the supraspinatus primarily (0°–15°) and then by the deltoid. From about 30° to 120°, both the glenohumeral joint and the scapula are moving, such that for every 3° of abduction, 2° are contributed by glenohumeral movement and 1° by scapular rotation. From 120° to 180°, abduction results exclusively from rotation of the scapula. Pain during upper arm dropping from full abduction is also typical of supraspinatus tendonitis.

357 A: Adrenal carcinoma

Hirsutism outside of the perimenarchal period, rapid progression of hirsutism, or signs of Cushing's syndrome or virilisation should indicate the possibility of an ovarian or adrenal neoplasm. Diagnostic testing should examine levels of serum testosterone, 17–hydroxyprogesterone, and DHEA-S (dehydroepiandrosterone sulphate). Levels of serum testosterone greater than 200 mg/dl (6.94 mmol/l) and/or DHEA-S greater than 700 μg/dl (24.3 μmol/l) in women are strongly indicative of virilising tumours. In patients with hirsutism of peripubertal onset and slow progression, regular menses, otherwise normal physical examination and no virilisation, the likelihood of an underlying neoplasm is small. Full hormonal investigation is usually warranted only in those patients with rapid progression of hirsutism, abrupt symptom onset or virilisation.

358 E: Venlafaxine works best in patients with loss of appetite as the main feature

When patients take prescribed antidepressants as directed, most can expect to feel better in one to three months. Patients who respond to treatment should be treated for 6–12 months from the day when they felt like they used to feel. Both elderly patients who have had one episode of depression and those who have had two or more previous episodes should take antidepressants indefinitely because the risk of relapse may be more than 80%.

For patients who do not respond to two or more trials of antidepressants, referral for augmentation with other psychiatric agents or treatment with electroconvulsive therapy is indicated. Psychotherapy, when available, remains a good addition to the treatment regimen. Maintaining an effective system for psychotherapy referral may also increase a patient's chances of feeling better and reduce the risk of relapse. It is important to keep in mind that the suicide risk may increase if a patient feels a boost in energy before achieving relief from hopelessness and suicidal thinking. This risk is also high if antidepressant therapy is stopped prematurely and negative thinking returns quickly. For those with symptoms of psychomotor retardation, one of the more activating antidepressants (eg fluoxetine, venlafaxine, bupropion) might be a good choice, while in those patients in great need of sleep, therapy with mirtazapine, nefazodone, paroxetine or fluvoxamine may be considered. Sertraline and citalopram cause little agitation or sedation and remain good middle-of-the-road choices. Mirtazapine and paroxetine are good choices for patients who can benefit from a stimulated appetite. Fluoxetine, venlafaxine and bupropion are good choices for patients who have hyperphagia or who are wary of possible weight gain.

359   C: Mixed connective tissue disease

This is a rheumatic disease syndrome characterised by overlapping clinical features of SLE, scleroderma, polymyositis or dermatomyositis, and rheumatoid arthritis and by very high titres of circulating antinuclear antibody to a nuclear ribonucleoprotein (RNP) antigen. The typical clinical syndrome is characterised by Raynaud's phenomenon, polyarthralgia or arthritis, swollen hands, inflammatory proximal myopathy, oesophageal hypomotility and pulmonary disease. Almost all patients have high titres (often > 1:1000) of fluorescent ANA that produce a speckled pattern. Immunodiffusion can confirm that antibody to RNP is present. High titres of antibody to RNP usually persist for years but they may decline significantly or become undetectable in patients in prolonged remission.

360   A: Hypertrophic cardiomyopathy

Although the overall population of athletes is at generally low risk for sudden death, a number of largely congenital but clinically unsuspected cardiovascular diseases have been causally linked to sudden death in young trained athletes, usually in association with physical exertion. In large autopsy-based surveys of populations of athletes, hypertrophic cardiomyopathy has been the single most common cardiovascular cause of sudden death. Ventricular tachyarrhythmia is the most probable cause of sudden death in this disorder. All the other options are possible causes of sudden death in athletes but they are less common. Tall R waves might indicate left ventricular hypertrophy secondary to aortic stenosis or hypertrophic cardiomyopathy, the latter a far more common cause of sudden death in athletes than the former.

361 E: Bradycardia
Neuroleptic malignant syndrome is a rare but potentially life-threatening complication of neuroleptic therapy. It consists of mental state changes, including confusion and mutism as well as physical abnormalities. Autonomic dysfunction, including elevated or labile blood pressure, tachycardia, hyperpyrexia and diaphoresis can occur, as well as dysphagia, tremor, rigidity and incontinence. Treatment varies, depending on the severity of presentation, but always includes the cessation of antipsychotic therapy.

362 C: *Haemophilus influenzae*
The picture is typical of aseptic meningitis. *Haemophilus influenzae* will cause bacterial meningitis. The WBC count in bacterial infection is typically greater than 1000 cells/mm³ with a predominance of neutrophils. A lower count or a lymphocytic predominance is found particularly in meningitis caused by *Listeria monocytogenes* or in bacterial meningitis that has been partially treated. The glucose levels and the ratio of CSF to serum glucose level are usually decreased and the CSF protein level is characteristically elevated. Lyme meningitis, tuberculous meningitis and *Mycoplasma pneumoniae* meningitis often present with an aseptic meningitis picture.

363 D: Gustatory hallucinations
Psychosis is defined as the presence of delusions, hallucinations and specific abnormalities of behaviour, such as catatonia, severe psychomotor retardation or overactivity. Autochthonous (primary) delusions are first-rank symptoms of schizophrenia. Hallucinations of any modality – including gustatory (taste) – are a feature of psychosis. Hypnogogic hallucinations are an exception as they refer specifically to auditory hallucinations experienced as one drifts to sleep. Echopraxia is a feature of cognitive impairment. Tardive dyskinesia may be a result of long-term antipsychotic medication, but does not indicate current psychosis. Disorientation is the hallmark of acute confusional state.

364 E: Clindamycin
Many drugs, such as certain non-steroidal anti-inflammatory drugs (particularly phenylbutazone, which is now rarely used), chloramphenicol, gold, sulphonamides and nifedipine are known to cause pancytopenia/aplastic anaemia. When due to phenylbutazone it usually occurs after prolonged treatment. Similarly, gold-induced pancytopenia typically occurs in patients who have received a total

dose of 200–450 mg and it is usually severe and often irreversible. Felbamate, an antiepileptic medication, has been associated with a number of cases of pancytopenia in the last few years.

365 A: Munchausen's syndrome
Brain scans in Alzheimer's disease may show cerebral atrophy, particularly in temporal lobe structures. Pick's disease may show bilateral atrophy of frontal lobes. In Huntington's disease there is atrophy of the caudate and frontotemporal regions. In schizophrenia the most common finding is enlargement of the lateral ventricles. Studies in depressive disorders have also shown temporal lobe changes. In elderly depressives white matter hyperintensities have been reported.

366 D: Single palmar crease
Fragile X syndrome is the second commonest cause of mental retardation in males. Clinical features include prognathism, hypertelorism, macro-orchidism and a single palmar crease. Learning difficulties accompanied by an absence of secondary male sexual characteristics is the picture associated with Klinefelter's syndrome. Strabismus occurs more frequently in Down's syndrome.

367 D: Hyperthyroidism
Depressive disorders occur more commonly than by chance in Addison's disease, Cushing's syndrome, hyperparathyroidism and hypothyroidism. Hyperthyroidism is more associated with anxiety.

368 C: Alcohol withdrawal delirium
Alcohol withdrawal delirium occurs when a person who uses alcohol excessively suddenly stops the alcohol use. Clinical manifestations include agitation, global confusion, disorientation, hallucinations, fever and autonomic hyperactivity (tachycardia and hypertension). Postoperative and orthopaedic trauma patients are cases were alcohol withdrawal delirium might be missed and attributed to alternative co-morbidity. Delayed recognition and treatment can lead to a complicated and extended hospital course. Alcohol withdrawal delirium occurs three to ten days after the last drink, which coincided here with the third postoperative day. The patient is often recovering well in the first 48 hours but a rapid and progressive decline ensues with no evidence of wound or abdominal cavity infection nor any obvious features of respiratory, cardiovascular or renal function disorder. A high index of suspicion is warranted. Deranged liver function tests and raised GGT might

give a clue to the possible cause of this mental change. Post-anaesthesia delirium usually manifests in the immediate postoperative period. Subdural haematoma is often associated with localising neurological signs.

369   C: Dopamine D$_2$

These medications have a variety of pharmacological actions. Their ability to block the dopamine (D$_2$) receptor in the mesolimbic system reduces positive symptoms of psychosis. The D$_2$ blockade in the nigrostriatal pathway causes extrapyramidal symptoms, which include drug-induced parkinsonism, akathisia, acute dystonia and tardive dyskinesia. The D$_2$-receptor blockade in the tuberoinfundibular pathway increases serum levels of prolactin, which may present clinically as breast tenderness, galactorrhoea or erectile dysfunction. Younger patients may present with amenorrhoea

370   B: Benzatropine 2 mg intravenously or intramuscularly

This is most likely to be an acute dystonic reaction to the metoclopromide. Dystonias are idiosyncratic drug reactions that involve acute involuntary muscle movements and spasms. Acute dystonia as an adverse effect of dopamine antagonists such as antipsychotic drugs (phenothiazines) and the anti-emetic drug metoclopromide affects about 2% of patients. It occurs abruptly and early in the treatment. Males, young adults and children are more susceptible. Although any muscle group in the body can be involved, the commonest manifestations are torticollis, facial grimacing and opisthotonos. The treatment is to discontinue the offending agent. Intravenous or intramuscular anticholinergics (eg benzatropine 2 mg) should be used. Diphenhydramine 50 mg either intramuscularly or intravenously is also effective. Improvement generally occurs within seconds or within 15–30 minutes. These doses can be repeated in 30 minutes. Even if the agent is discontinued, oral treatment with either agent should be continued orally for 24–48 hours, because symptoms can recur for up to two weeks following cessation of the offending drug.

371   E: Tuberculin skin test

The lesions in the mouth are typical of aphthous ulcers, which could be either primary or secondary. The secondary form is often associated with one of the following conditions: rheumatoid diseases including Behçet's disease, Reiter's syndrome and lupus erythematosus, coeliac disease, Crohn's disease, ulcerative colitis and malabsorption syndromes, and adverse drug reactions (eg erythema multiforme). Tuberculosis is a rare cause of mucous membrane (oral cavity and conjunctiva) ulceration. The ulcers, when they do develop, are often single and are usually larger than aphthous ulcers.

372 C: Squamous cell carcinoma

Squamous cell carcinoma arises in the proximal portions of the tracheobronchial tree in 60–80% of cases. Central and peripheral squamous cell carcinoma may show extensive central necrosis with resulting cavitation. A cavitating mass close to the right hilum is most likely be squamous cell carcinoma of the bronchus. Furthermore, due to production of parathyroid hormone-related peptide (PTHrP), as seen most frequently with tumours of squamous cell histology. Most adenocarcinomas are peripheral in location. Although small cell carcinomas are mostly of central origin, hypercalcaemia, when present, is usually secondary to bone metastasis and not associated with increased levels of PTHrP.

373 D: Blood eosinophilia

The most direct assessment of the impact of airflow obstruction on ventilation is measurement of arterial blood gases. Hypoxaemia severe enough to present with clinical cyanosis indicates severe asthma and status asthmaticus. Far more important is the arterial Pco_2. Respiratory drive is almost invariably increased in acute asthma, resulting in hyperventilation and a correspondingly decreased $Paco_2$. Thus, an elevated or even normal $Paco_2$ indicates that airway narrowing is so severe that the ventilatory demands of the respiratory centre cannot be met. Respiratory failure can then develop rapidly with any further bronchoconstriction or respiratory muscle fatigue. A peak flow below 120 l/minute or an FEV_1 below 1.0 litre indicates severe obstruction in all but unusually small adults. Tachycardia >120 bpm and pulusus paradoxicus > 15 mmHg are important indices of severe asthma. The presence of blood eosinophilia in an asthmatic patient is highly suggestive of atopy as an underlying cause of the asthma. It is not a marker of severe disease.

374 A: Resting $Paco_2$ of 8 kPa

This patient is suffering from interstitial lung disease secondary to a connective tissue disorder (systemic sclerosis). Most of the interstitial disorders have a restrictive defect with reductions in total lung capacity (TLC), functional residual capacity (FRC) and residual volume (RV). Flow rates are decreased (FEV_1 and FVC) but the changes are in proportion to the decreased lung volumes – the FEV_1/FVC ratio is therefore usually normal or increased. The reductions in lung volumes become more pronounced as lung stiffness worsens with disease progression. A reduction in the diffusion capacity (DLCO) is a commonly found in interstitial lung diseases. The decrease in DLCO is due in part to effacement of the alveolar capillary units but also more importantly, to the extent of mismatching of ventilation and perfusion of the alveoli. The severity of the DLCO reduction does not correlate well with disease stage. The blood gases often reveal evidence of hypoxia with a low PaO_2, which declines further with exercise. The $PaCO_2$ is usually normal and even decreases further with exercise and hyperventilation.

375 B: The patient says the thoughts are stupid and tries not to think them

Obsessional phenomena are recurrent intrusive thoughts, impulses or images that the patient accepts are their own (ie arising internally) but are perceived as senseless and therefore unwanted and resisted. Delusional beliefs are held with subjective certainty, and so are not resisted. The importance of delineating obsessional from psychotic phenomena is important as the risk to the baby is far greater with the latter. Believing the thoughts are not hers may suggest thought insertion; a first rank symptom of schizophrenia.

376 B: *Pneumocystis carinii* pneumonia

Bacterial pneumonia (typical or atypical) is often associated with pleural effusion. In *Mycoplasma pneumoniae* pneumonia pleural effusions can be seen in up to 20% of patients when lateral decubitus films are performed. Fungal and parasitic chest infections are also known to be associated with pleural effusion. However, the most common radiographic abnormalities in *Pneumocystis carinii* pneumonia are diffuse bilateral interstitial or alveolar infiltrates. Less common presentations include pneumothoraces, and lobar or segmental infiltrates. Pleural effusions are rarely encountered in *Pneumocystis carinii* pneumonia.

377 C: Half the sons will be affected

Becker's muscular dystrophy is an X-linked recessive inherited disorder. A family history of similarly affected maternal uncles assists the clinician with confirming a diagnosis of Becker's muscular dystrophy.

X-linked recessive disease is characterised by the following:

- A heterozygous female will transmit the disease to half of her sons
- Half the daughters of a heterozygous mother will be carriers.

378   D: Korsakoff's psychosis

Basic cognitive examination can be useful in distinguishing organic from functional mental illness. Korsakoff's psychosis is an amnesic syndrome, characterised in particular by impaired recent memory. As a consequence there is disorientation in time. Established dementia and delirium are also associated with temporal disorientation. Acute schizophrenia or other mood disorders are not associated with disorientation to time.

379   E: Mumps virus

The CSF picture is suggestive of viral meningitis. Worldwide causes of viral meningitis include enteroviruses, mumps virus, measles virus, varicella zoster virus and human immunodeficiency virus. The majority (over 80%) of all cases are caused by enteroviruses, followed by the mumps virus. Pleocytosis with blood WBC counts in the range of 50 to > 1000 x 10^9/l has been reported in viral meningitis. Mononuclear cell predominance is the rule; CSF protein level is usually only slightly elevated; and the glucose level is normal in most cases. Bacterial meningitis has a much higher cell count and a predominance of neutrophils in the cell differential count. The protein is elevated and the glucose is usually low. Non-bacterial meningitis, such as tuberculous meningitis, is an important cause of aseptic meningitis. It has a very similar CSF picture to viral meningitis but the glucose levels are very low and the protein is significantly higher.

380   E: Weight loss

Irritable bowel syndrome is a functional gastrointestinal syndrome characterised by chronic abdominal pain and altered bowel habits in the absence of any organic cause. It is the most commonly diagnosed gastrointestinal condition. Pain associated with malnutrition or weight loss should prompt an investigation for organic disease.

381   A: Rapid urease test

The diagnosis of *Helicobacter pylori* infection can usually be established during endoscopy by one of three methods: biopsy urease test, histology and, less commonly, bacterial culture. When endoscopy is indicated, the test of first choice is a urease test on an antral biopsy. Rapid urease testing is a colorimetric test based on the ability of *H. pylori* to produce urease and it provides rapid testing at the time of biopsy. Because of the desire to know a patient's *H. pylori* status before discharge from the endoscopy suite, specialised urea membrane kits have been designed specifically to give a result within one hour. If a biopsy urease test is negative, *H. pylori* infection may be diagnosed by histology or serology. Serology and a breath test are usually done in patients in whom endoscopy is not planned.

382 A: It is asymptomatic in most cases

Approximately 1% of patients with Barrett's oesophagus per year progress to carcinoma. Barrett's oesophagus *per se* is usually asymptomatic. It is usually recognised as an incidental finding at endoscopy. It consists of a columnar-lined distal oesophagus due to intestinal metaplasia of the distal oesophageal mucosa. It is an acquired condition due to gastro-oesophageal reflux. It is not related to *Helicobacter pylori* infection.

383 C: It is secreted by special cells in the parathyroid gland

Calcitonin is a polypeptide of 32 amino acids. The thyroid cells in which it is synthesised have receptors that bind calcium ions (Ca^{2+}) circulating in the blood. These cells monitor the level of circulating Ca^{2+}. A rise in its level stimulates the cells to release calcitonin. Bone cells respond by removing Ca^{2+} from the blood and storing it in the bone; kidney cells respond by increasing the excretion of Ca^{2+}. Both these types of cells have surface receptors for calcitonin. Because it promotes the transfer of Ca^{2+} to bones, calcitonin has been examined as a possible treatment for osteoporosis. Being a polypeptide, calcitonin cannot be given by mouth (it would be digested) and giving by injection is not appealing. However, inhaling calcitonin appears to be an effective way to get therapeutic levels of the hormone into the bloodstream. A synthetic version of calcitonin is now available as a nasal spray.

384 C: Fluoride

Wrist fracture may be an early indication of the presence of osteoporosis and should prompt further investigations for underlying osteoporosis. This patient does have osteoporosis as confirmed on the DEXA scan. Treatment should be initiated as soon as possible to prevent future fractures in other vulnerable sites such as the hip and spine.

Although fluoride seems to improve bone mineral density (BMD), its ability to change fracture rates has been minimal. Controlled data clearly show that all three bisphosphonates increase bone mineral density at the spine and hip in a dose-dependent manner. Although no clinical trials have focused on hip fracture as a primary outcome, most studies have shown that oestrogen replacement has improved BMD. Calcitonin has been shown to have positive effects on BMD in the vertebral spine; the data are less clear for the hip. Nasal calcitonin and selective oestrogen-receptor modulators (SERMs) are standard treatments for osteoporosis. More recently, parathyroid hormone has been approved as an effective treatment for osteoporosis.

385 C: Respiratory arrest

Patients who are in acute respiratory distress and are at risk of requiring intubation should be selected for non-invasive ventilation if they have a reversible cause of acute respiratory failure. Non-invasive positive-pressure ventilation (NPPV) decreases the work of breathing and thereby improves alveolar ventilation while simultaneously resting the respiratory musculature. NPPV is delivered by a nasal or face mask, therefore eliminating the need for intubation or tracheostomy. NPPV can be given by a volume ventilator, a pressure-controlled ventilator, a bi-level positive airway pressure (BiPAP or bi-level ventilator) device, or a continuous positive airway pressure (CPAP) device. Volume ventilators are often not tolerated because they generate high inspiratory pressures that result in discomfort and mouth leaks. NPPV delivers a set pressure for each breath (with a bi-level or standard ventilator in the pressure-support mode). Although positive-pressure support is usually well tolerated by patients, mouth leaks or other difficulties are sometimes encountered. BiPAP ventilators provide continuous high-flow positive airway pressure that cycles between a high positive pressure and a lower positive pressure. NPPV may be used as an intermittent mode of assistance depending on the patient's clinical situation. Instantaneous and continuous support is given to patients in acute respiratory distress. As the underlying condition improves, ventilator-free periods are increased as tolerated, and support is discontinued when the patient is deemed stable. In most studies, the duration of NPPV use in patients with acute on chronic respiratory failure averages at 6–18 hours. The total duration of ventilator use varies with the underlying disease: approximately six hours in acute pulmonary oedema and more than two days for COPD exacerbations.

Guidelines for the use of NPPV in patients with acute respiratory failure:

- Blood gas findings
  Partial pressure of carbon dioxide in arterial blood > 6 kPa
  pH < 7.35 but > 7.10
  PaO_2 < 6 kPa
- Clinical inclusion criteria:
  Signs or symptoms of acute respiratory distress
  Moderate to severe dyspnoea (increased over usual)
  Respiratory rate greater than 24/minute
  Accessory muscle use
  Abdominal paradox
- Diagnosis (type of patients):
  COPD exacerbation
  Acute pulmonary oedema
  Pneumonia
- Contraindications:
  Respiratory arrest (intubation and mechanical ventilation should
  be introduced without delay).

386 E: Meningitis

Cytomegalovirus (CMV) is a member of the herpesvirus family and shares with other herpesviruses the capacity to remain latent after recovery from an acute infection. A low degree of viral persistence, tightly controlled by immune surveillance, may be present in infected cells. Immunosuppression after transplantation will result in enhanced viral replication and eventually in the development of CMV infection or disease. CMV infection exhibits a wide range of clinical manifestations, from asymptomatic infection to severe or lethal CMV disease. Patients who develop CMV disease can be further subdivided into those with and those without organ involvement. Symptomatic infection without documentation of organ involvement is usually called 'viral syndrome' (fever, leukopenia, thrombocytopenia and other constitutional symptoms, such as malaise and arthralgias). Organ involvement with CMV correlates with the organ transplanted. This means that CMV hepatitis occurs more frequently in liver transplant recipients and CMV pancreatitis in pancreas transplant recipients. Pneumonitis results in fever, dyspnoea and cough, with findings of hypoxaemia and pulmonary infiltrates.

The more severe form of digestive tract disease is hepatitis. Serious CMV hepatitis requiring intensive therapy is not uncommon in liver transplant patients and it typically manifests as elevated concentrations of γ-glutamyltransferase and alkaline phosphatase in addition to increased levels of transaminases. A high index of suspicion of CMV colitis should be maintained in any transplant patient who presents with lower gastrointestinal bleeding in the first four months after transplantation. CMV retinitis is infrequent in this population and it usually presents more than six months after transplantation. Patients may be asymptomatic or may experience blurring of vision, scotomata or decreased visual acuity. The diagnosis is made fundoscopically. CMV encephalitis and transverse myelitis are recognised but are relatively rare. CMV meningitis is not reported in such patients.

387 C: Zidovudine therapy should be initiated if there is any evidence of seroconversion

Blood-borne diseases that could be transmitted by such an injury include human immunodeficiency virus (HIV), hepatitis B (HBV) and hepatitis C (HCV). The risk of HIV transmission following needlestick injury involving contaminated blood is estimated to be about 0.4%. Her risk of contracting HIV infection is low and much less than for hepatitis B and C. If the source patient is HIV-positive or is of unknown status, the injured person should be encouraged to undergo baseline HIV testing. Counselling and consent are important in this situation. The injured person should be followed up for at least six months. Blood should be taken soon after the injury and also at six months after exposure. There is evidence that the use of zidovudine prophylaxis reduces the risk of transmission by about 80%. Prophylaxis should be started, ideally within 1–2 hours of exposure. Seroconversion may occur weeks to months later. It is advisable that this nurse avoids getting pregnant and sex should be protected from the time of exposure until the second HIV test is negative at the end of the six months. Strict confidentiality of the HIV status of patients and staff must be observed.

388 B: Hodgkin's disease

Hodgkin's disease has been principally described in association with minimal-change nephropathy and rarely with membranous glomerulonephritis.

389 A: Female gender

The risk of developing DVT begins to increase statistically at the age of 40. The risk of DVT is not predicted independently by gender. Some risk factors (pregnancy, hormone replacement therapy) are gender-specific and may account for the diagnosis being more common among women in study populations. Obesity is an independent predictor of the likelihood of DVT probably because of lower extremity venous hypertension. Even though this patient has stopped smoking, her risk of DVT is independently elevated above that of a lifelong non-smoker.

390   B: Citalopram

These antidepressants are probably equally effective, except venlafaxine which may have an advantage in terms of speed of onset and rates of improvement. Four issues should be considered here:

- the propensity of some antidepressants (especially tricyclics and venlafaxine) to exacerbate cardiovascular disease (heart failure and conduction defects)
- the risk of affecting glycaemic control (fluoxetine)
- the risk of interactions with other medication (especially fluoxetine/ venlafaxine and warfarin
- toxicity in overdose (amitriptyline and dothiepin).

On balance, citalopram is probably the best choice.

391   A: Facial lesions

Patients should be taught to be aware of the following warning signs in any naevus or 'mole': the development of itching, burning, swelling or pain in a pre-existing mole; the development of raised areas in a previously flat lesion; a change in the consistency of a lesion; a change in surface characteristics, such as bleeding, scaling, ulceration, or crusting; and the development of satellite lesions. Although malignant melanomas are often seen on the trunk there is no true correlation between the site of the mole and its tendency to become malignant. New moles in older adults should be reported to the doctor and monitored carefully.

392   D: Allopurinol

Allopurinol is a xanthine oxidase inhibitor that inhibits uric acid formation and therefore lowers its level in the body. Indometacin, colchicine and prednisolone are considered effective treatments for acute gout but they have no hypouricaemic effects. Low-dose aspirin competes with renal uric acid excretion and increases uric acid levels in serum.

393   A: He should hold the stick in the left hand

A stick should be held on the side opposite the arthritic knee. Valgus deformity is more common in rheumatoid arthritis while varus (bow-legged) deformity is more common with osteoarthritis. Synovial fluid collection in the joint is also common in degenerative diseases such as osteoarthritis. The fluid volume varies and could reach 100 ml. A Baker's cyst is a manifestation of knee arthritis, regardless of the underlying pathology.

394 E: Neuropathic joint disease

This patient's high glucose concentration and absent ankle tendon reflex suggests that he is apparently suffering from diabetic neuropathy. This has been complicated by neuropathic joint disease (osteoarthropathy) which can be defined as bone and joint changes that occur secondary to loss of sensation. Charcot first described the relationship between loss of sensation and arthropathy in 1868. The radiographic changes include destruction of articular surfaces, opaque subchondral bones, joint debris (loose bodies), deformity and dislocation. Neuropathic arthropathy poses a special problem in imaging when it is associated with a soft tissue infection.

The pathophysiology of neuropathic arthropathy is debatable. The general consensus is that the loss of proprioception and deep sensation leads to recurrent trauma, which ultimately leads to progressive destruction, degeneration and disorganisation of the joint. Another theory postulates that a neurally mediated vascular reflex results in hyperaemia, which can cause osteoclastic bone resorption. Causes of neuropathic arthropathy include diabetes, syphilis, syringomyelia and leprosy.

395 C: Right-sided hemiplegia

In most reports, 47–76% of patients achieve partial or total independence in performance of activities of daily living (ADL). The strongest predictors of poor physical recovery occur in the first 24 hours:

- Total flaccid paralysis of the arm and leg
- Conjugate gaze palsy (patient cannot spontaneously move his eyes towards his paralysed limbs because of damage to the centre for conjugate eye movements)
- Non-dominant hemiplegia and neglect (left-side hemiplegia in right-handed patients)
- Reduced level of consciousness
- Incontinence
- Co-morbidity.

Age in itself does not influence the gross neurological aspects of stroke, but older age is associated with co-morbidity and with poorer recovery in ability to perform the activities of daily living.

396 B: Son's children 0%; daughter's children 100%

At fertilisation all mitochondria in the zygote come from the oocyte and so both mtDNA and most mtDNA-related diseases are maternally inherited.

397 E: Osteonecrosis

Osteonecrosis (avascular necrosis of bone) occurs in 14% of patients with systemic lupus erythematosus. It most commonly affects the hip joints. Early detection requires magnetic resonance imaging. Core decompression of bone is an effective treatment in the early stages of the disease. The major risk factors for osteonecrosis include a prednisolone dosage greater than 20 mg per day for one month or longer, and the presence of Raynaud's disease, nephritis or vasculitis. Flare-up of lupus arthropathy is usually polyarticular. The course of septic arthritis is more dramatic and the patient would seek attention within a few days. Her age is against a diagnosis of osteoarthritis.

398 A: The raised ESR rules out fibromyalgia as a possible diagnosis

Polymyalgia rheumatica (PMR) is a chroninc inflammatory condition characterised by stiffness and aching at the shoulder girdle and the pelvic and limb girdles. The symptoms are worse in the morning. There are a few patients who may develop giant cell arteritis with the development of temporal-distribution headaches. The ESR and C-reactive protein are classically elevated, although a small percentage of patients may have a normal test. Prednisolone remains the mainstay of therapy.

Fibromyalgia is best described as a syndrome with pain 'all over' and characterised by tender points in a certain distribution such as the neck, trapezius, and supraspinatus muscle regions. Other areas include the second anterior rib, lateral epicondyle and the greater trochanter. The lower back and medial aspect of the knee are areas where tender spots are also identified in patients with fibromyalgia. All these tender points are symmetrical or bilateral. Fibromyalgia is not an inflammatory disorder and therefore the ESR is typically normal and it does not predispose to giant cell arteritis.

PMR and fibromyalgia are chronic disorders characterised by remissions and relapses that can go on for many years.

399 C: Sensitivity can be calculated from data on just those subjects having the gold standard diagnosis of prostate cancer

Sensitivity is the percentage (or proportion) of subjects who are 'true positives' (having prostate cancer) who are also 'test positive' ie

100% × (no. of subjects who truly have prostate cancer and also test positive)/(number of subjects who truly have prostate cancer).

A is not appropriate because sensitivity is not directly linked to specificity. A test can have high sensitivity and low specificity.

B is inappropriate because sensitivity is not affected by prevalence.

C is correct because the formula for sensitivity (see above) requires data from those with 'true' prostate cancer alone.

D is incorrect because if sensitivity were 100% then this would indicate that there would be no false negative results with the test.

E is incorrect because the addition of sensitivity and specificity values is not constrained to equal 100%.

400 D: Red cell mass

The raised haemoglobin levels in a middle-aged man who has hypertension and splenomegaly on physical examination should alert you to the possibility of polycythaemia rubra vera (PRV). The pathophysiology of PRV is a result of a myeloproliferative disorder causing erythroid hyperplasia independant of raised cirulating erythropoietin. In addition to a raised haemoglobin and red cell count, the white cells are also increased in 70% and the platelets in 50%, and physical examination may demonstrate a palpable spleen. A high red cell mass will confirm the diagnosis.

In contrast, secondary polycythaemia is due to raised levels of circulating erythropoietin, either due to a physiological response (eg living at high altitude, chronic lung disease or cyanotic heart disease) or to inappropriate secretion of erythropoietin from various sources (renal carcinoma or hepatoma). In this condition, although the red cell mass is also high, the white cells and platelets are unaffected and the spleen is not palpable.

Gaissbock's syndrome (pseudopolycythaemia) occurs in middle-aged men who are usually obese and have a smoking history. In this case the red cell mass is normal but the plasma volume is reduced.

Index

Locators are question/answer number